STUDIES
IN HISTORY OF
BIOLOGY

STUDIES
IN HISTORY OF
BIOLOGY

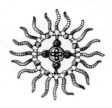

1

William Coleman
and Camille Limoges
Editors

The Johns Hopkins University Press
BALTIMORE AND LONDON

The Johns Hopkins University Press, Baltimore, Maryland 21218
The Johns Hopkins Press Ltd., London

Library of Congress Catalog Card Number 76–47139
ISBN 0–8018–1862–1
Library of Congress Cataloging in Publication data will be found on the last printed page of this book.

Contributors wishing to publish in *Studies in History of Biology* are invited to communicate with either of the editors:

WILLIAM COLEMAN, Department of the History of Science, The Johns Hopkins University, Baltimore, Maryland 21218 USA

CAMILLE LIMOGES, Institut d'Histoire et de Sociopolitique des Sciences, Université de Montréal, C.P. 6128, Montreal H3C 3J7, Québec, Canada

*To the memory
of our friend and fellow historian*
Charles A. Culotta

Contents

STUDIES
IN HISTORY OF
BIOLOGY

The Gene as Catalyst;
The Gene as Organism

Arnold W. Ravin

I. Introduction

From very early times the problems of heredity and development have been intertwined. In explaining how a new organism is brought into being, the investigator of living things had to account as well for the phenomenon of resemblance between offspring and parents. Conversely, if one began with the question of resemblance, such resemblances as were observed had to come about within the context of the developing organism. In short, explanations of heredity and development had to be compatible even when not completely unified.

Today the biologist makes the connection between heredity and development in a relatively untroubled way. Molecular models of gene action make it easy for him to distinguish between *transmission* of a reproducible material that makes possible the development of certain characters in the organism and the actual *expression* or realization of those characters in the course of a complex series of events he calls development. Even if a satisfactory understanding of the events underlying expression is not yet at hand, the modern developmental biologist hardly doubts that the ultimate understanding will involve some selective expression (the "turning on" and "off") of components of the genotype. The distinction between a reproducible genetic material and its expression, so taken for granted by the modern student, was not always apparent to earlier students of life. The distinction has indeed become central to our current understanding of the relation between heredity and development, and a historic appraisal of its origin is merited. In offering such an appraisal, this article will show that the important conception of a genetic material whose reproduction is independent of its expression (in the develop-

Arnold W. Ravin, Department of Biology and Committee of Conceptual Foundations of Science, University of Chicago.

mental sense of determining adult body characters) was a product of a very early convergence of genetics and biochemistry at the beginning of the twentieth century. Like most ideas at their inception, this one was associated with others that are now regarded as erroneous. Nevertheless, the fundamental notion was lifted from its context, and when associated with a combination of other ideas already existing in the writings of various biologists, it served to bring more closely together the then separate sciences of heredity and development. It also came to play an influential role in framing new conceptions of organism and of the origin of life itself.

Metaphysical and other preconceptions marked the history of this idea. Indeed, to trace the notion of a distinction between reproducible material and its developmental expression, it will be useful to sketch the nineteenth-century background, for it was out of the hope of settling the raging contest between material, preformationist, and vitalistic, epigenetic theories that the notion was born.

II. Background

Since the pre-Socratic philosophers until fairly recent times, theories of development and heredity have swung between two contrasting views often referred to as preformation and epigenesis. Preformationists generally postulated a material link between parents and offspring and a correspondence between elements of the parental contribution and elements of the parental body organization. Over the years, preformationists differed in their ways of specifying the exact nature of this correspondence—from supposing, on the one hand, that the new organism is literally all there at the outset, however miniature, in the parental contribution to supposing, on the other hand, that only the "germ" of the adult organization exists prior to development that consists in elaboration upon this basic, germinal plan. Yet they agreed at least that the characters by which we describe organisms and by means of which resemblances are observed are somehow those of the material elements transmitted from generation to generation.

The preformationist view of development and heredity thus ran counter to an argument set forth by Aristotle, which is as compelling today as when first uttered. Realizing that the organism is a coherent, harmoniously working assemblage of parts, and distinguishing between nonuniform parts (hands, feet, etc.), which are composed of a variety of apparently homogeneous, uniform parts (sinews, hair, bone, etc.), which are in turn composed of the elements (fire, air, water, and earth), Aristotle argued as follows:

> The non-uniform parts are constructed out of uniform parts assembled together. . . .
> Now flesh and bones, we should agree, are constructed out of fire and the like

substances, which means that the semen would be drawn from the elements only, for how can it possibly be drawn from the assemblage of them? And yet without this assemblage the parts would not have the resemblance, so if there is something which sets to work later on to bring the assemblage about, then surely this something, and not the drawing of the semen from the whole of the [parent's] body, will be the cause of this resemblance?[1]

Resemblance, Aristotle reminds us, resides in organizational matters, and if the *entire* adult organization does not exist in the semen—as seemed unlikely to Aristotle—something must work to bring the adult arrangement into being. For Aristotle this thing could not be material; rather it was a nonmaterial formative agency contributed by the male parent, working upon the matter supplied by the female parent in much the same way as a sculptor shapes clay by means of a preexisting form (except that in the developing organism the sculptor and the form are combined). Moreover, the formative agency worked in conjunction with another causal factor (the final cause), which acted for the sake of generating a new individual. To the extent that Aristotle's formative agency and final cause were nonmaterial, they became the basis of nonmaterial, vitalistic philosophies that waxed and waned in subsequent centuries. To the extent that in Aristotle's view of generation the entire adult body organization was not present in the semen and must be brought about through a series of events, it became the basis of epigenetic theories starting but not ending with Harvey.[2] But the vitalistic and the epigenetic aspects of "Aristotelian" theory were not necessarily wedded indissolubly to each other, and they could be, as they eventually were, separated by accepting the latter without the former.

In the nineteenth century, preformationist and vitalistic doctrines reached a stage of serious confrontation once it was realized that cells constituted the maternal and paternal contributions to the individual of the next generation. It was the sperm (or pollen) and egg that united to give rise to the zygote, or first cell of the new individual. Yet the adult individual came to contain many hundreds to millions of cells (depending upon the species), and these cells became morphologically and functionally differentiated, yet organized at every stage of development to achieve an integrated, harmonious organism. Microscopic observation of the events transpiring during development revealed, therefore, complex alterations in cellular structure and intercellular organization; development was patently epigenetic and there was little further quarrel about that. But was it a material agency in the gametes that shaped the subsequent development of the embryonic organism, or was it something immaterial, no physical part of the cell, that did so?

A clear theoretical formulation in material terms was set forth by August Weismann in the latter part of the nineteenth century. His theory was developed in a series of essays written between 1883 and 1891[3] and presented in a more formal manner in his book, *The Germ Plasm* published in 1892.[4] Two principal themes ran through Weismann's thought, one concerning the possibility of the inheritance of acquired characters and the other dealing with the role of the nucleus in heredity and development. Certain versions of preformationism[5] had from quite early times, as Hippocrates[6] and Aristotle[7] both realized, implied inheritance of acquired characters, since modifications of the parental body organization ought to alter the parts composing it and so contribute altered components to the "seed." Darwin's model of pangenesis[8] was indeed a formal presentation of this idea within the context of nineteenth-century knowledge of cells and gametes.

Weismann rejected the notion of transmission of acquired characters as early as 1883 in his essay "On Heredity."[9] He started from the facts that each organism began its development from a single cell (the fertilized egg) and that this cell gave rise to the many cells of which the adult organism was comprised. Among the cellular descendants of the original cell, however, he made a distinction between those that constitute the body proper, or *soma*, and those that are the gametes, or *germ cells*, to be involved in initiating the next generation of organisms. Weismann found it impossible to imagine how changes in the soma could affect the material contained in the germ cells so as to cause corresponding changes to appear in the offspring. Apparently to Weismann, the embryological studies undertaken at the cellular level during the nineteenth century indicated that the germ cell was not formed gradually by the accretion of material contributions from somatic tissue, but rather was a product of the same divisions that gave rise to the soma and so became separated from the soma. If the soma was not the material source of the components of the germ cell, what then was?

Weismann was not about to abandon a material conception of heredity; he simply rejected one preformationist version of it. His writings give clear evidence that he was thinking in terms of a material substance contained in the germ cells, or *germ plasm*, that somehow directs the course of development. Weismann said, for example, that his "theory of the continuity of the germ plasm" (the notion that the germ cells were derived not from the soma, but from preexisting germ cells) was in fact "founded upon the idea that heredity is brought about by the transference from one generation to another, of a substance with a definite chemical, and above all, molecular constitution."[10] Moreover, this germ plasm, a material version of Aristotle's formative agency, was undoubtedly contained within the nucleus of the germ cell, and more specifically within the chromosomes. This view was argued persuasively in a series of essays that pointed out the significant role the chromosomes had been shown to play in cell division and gametogenesis by the cytologists Oscar Hertwig, Herman Fol, Charles van Beneden, and Eduard Strasburger, among others. "Thus the nuclear substance must be the sole bearer of hereditary tendencies.''[11] It acted so by sending molecular stimuli out into the cytoplasm, thereby impressing its specific character upon the cell.[12]

In order to account for the progressive differentiation of the somatic cells in the course of ontogeny, Weismann arrived at the idea that the germ plasm was actually transformed in exerting its control of development. This line of reasoning was revealed in such sentences as: ''. . . in each ontogeny, a part of the specific germ plasm is not *used up* in the construction of the offspring, but is reserved unchanged for the formation of the germ-cells of the following generation'' (italics mine).[13]

On the other hand, the somatic cells derive a transformed portion of the germ plasm, which becomes progressively diminished in quality in the course of differentiation of the somatic cells. ''This process would take place in a definitely ordered course. . . . and the determining and directing factor is simply and solely the nuclear substance. . . . which possesses such a molecular structure in the germ-cell that all such succeeding stages of its molecular structure in future nuclei must necessarily arise from it, as soon as the requisite external conditions are present.''[14] Two significant points were made in this argument. In the first place, the material germ plasm was consumed in the process of directing the development of the soma. Second, in the line connecting the germ cells of one generation with those of the next, there was no consumption of the germ plasm, but rather a reproduction of it. What cell division in the germ line was all about was the equitable distribution of chromosomal material—the germ plasm—which had been reproduced between divisions. That was what accounted for the similarity in number and size of the chromosomes in germ cells of succeeding generations of individuals of the same species, and it was what underlay the significance of the reduction divisions that occurred during oogenesis[15] and spermatogenesis.[16]

Of course, the continuity of the germ plasm was not absolute. Weismann concluded only that somatogenic variations, that is, changes produced by reaction of the body or soma, cannot produce chromosomal changes in the germ that will cause similar somatic variations in subsequent generations. ''It is impossible to assume the transmission of somatogenic variations in any theory which accepts the nuclear substance of the germ cells as germ plasm or 'hereditary substance;' for it is theoretically impossible to account for these variations no matter how ingeniously the theory is constructed.''[17] Consequently, ''all permanent—i.e., hereditary—variations of the body proceed from primary modifications of the constituents of the germ.''[18]

For Weismann, then, the germ plasm could not be reproduced and used to direct development *in the same cells*. He distributed these two functions between different cells. The two functions were not truly independent since they excluded each other. It is difficult to be certain how he arrived at this theory of somatic cell differentiation. He was aware of much cytological work with plant and animal cells, showing that the chromosomes of daughter cells appear similar in quantitative respects to each other and to those of the mother cell from which they arise by cell division. But, Weismann cautioned; "... we must not forget that we do not see the molecular structure of the nucleo-plasm but something which we can only look upon (when we remember how complex this molecular structure must be) as a very rough expression of its quantity . . . [its] division into two exactly equal parts would give us no proof of equality or inequality in [its] constitution. . . . We can only obtain proofs as to the quality of the molecular structure of the two halves by their effect on the bodies of the daughter-cells, and we know that these latter are frequently different in size and quality."[19] Therefore, he had to propose that, despite its apparent quantitative similarity, the chromosomal material is unequal in the somatic cells.

Like Watson and Crick's major contribution a century later, Weismann's work was primarily theoretical in nature, at least in the sense of being based hardly at all on his own observations and experiments. Nevertheless, like the Watson-Crick model of DNA structure, Weismann's theory of the continuity of the germ plasm had enormous impact. It influenced the thought of, among others, Wilhelm Roux and Theodore Boveri in Germany, William Bateson in England, and E. B. Wilson in the United States.

Yet Weismann's ideas were not without their detractors toward the close of the century. Among the most formidable of these were Hugo de Vries and Hans Driesch, no small theoreticians themselves. While de Vries attempted to save that part of Weismann's theory that postulated material units of heredity, Driesch sought to demolish it. Both attacked the theory, however, on the question of the consumption of the putatively directive germ plasm during development. The theoretical objection of de Vries is contained in his *In-tracelluläre Pangenesis* of 1889.[20] De Vries saw the phenomena of budding in plants and regeneration in animals as constituting difficulties for Weismann's notion, since in these cases new organs and even whole organisms appeared to arise out of somatic and not germ tissue. Hence, to retain the idea of a germ plasm made up of material entities, de Vries simply postulated that these units[21] could multiply in the nucleus and copies could enter the cytoplasm but remain latent. Like Weismann's germ plasm, de Vries's units, when active, were consumed by being directly converted into the various organelles of the cell. When inactive, they nevertheless retained the capacity for eventual use in forming cell constituents. This ingenious reconciliation of material units of heredity with the regulative capacity of the organism comes close to the modern version of gene action, except for the units themselves being the direct precursors of protoplasmic stuff. De Vries apparently abandoned this conception of development after his discovery of the Mendelian "laws," which indicated to him that the cell could contain at most two copies (maternal and paternal) of each hereditary determinant, and these copies had to be restricted to the nucleus. Thus, the excitement in the discovery of Mendelism was responsible for a temporary disappearance of the idea of *latency*; it was to be resurrected in a new form at a later time.

Hans Driesch, for his part, attempted to subject the notion of a consumed germ plasm to an experimental test. If this part of Weismann's theory were correct, embryonic cell divisions should soon make a mosaic of irreversibly determined cells apart from the few germ cells that conserved their hereditary substance. A disturbed arrangement of this mosaic ought not to result in a normal animal, nor should every cell upon isolation from the mosaic be capable of giving rise to a normal animal. Driesch's mentor, Wilhelm Roux, appeared to have confirmed this prediction when he obtained a half-embryo by killing one of the two cells resulting from the first cleavage division of the fertilized frog egg.[22] Yet the contrary was what Driesch's experiments on sea urchin embryos purported to show: isolated cells from the 4-cell embryonic stage were each capable of giving rise to a normal and complete, albeit small, larva.[23] Moreover, all cases of morphogenetic regulation, regeneration, and of adventitious growth in plants, were taken by Driesch as arguments against Weismann's scheme.

In apparently refuting that part of Weismann's theory bearing on consumption of the germ plasm during development, Driesch went much further to deny any *material* basis of heredity and development. His own theory, avowedly vitalistic, was drawn up in full array in the Gifford Lectures delivered before the University of Aberdeen in 1907, although it appeared in gradually maturing versions in earlier publications.[24] Driesch was impressed with the developing organism, to use his terms, as a harmonious, equipotential system: each of its cells or tissue types can give rise to any other, although each part is normally subjugated to undertake a more limited structural and functional role in the economy of the whole organism. The considerable power of the part to regulate itself depending upon its context could not be the work, according to him, of a material mechanism:

... an autonomy of life phenomena exists at least in some departments of individual morphogenesis, and probably in all of them; the real starting point of all morphogenesis cannot be regarded as a machine, nor can the real process of differentiation, in all cases where it is based upon systems of the harmonious equipotential type. There cannot be any sort of machine in the cell from which the individual originates, because this cell, including both its protoplasm and its nucleus, has undergone a long series of divisions, all resulting in equal products, and because a machine cannot be divided and in spite of that remain what it was. There cannot be, on the other hand, any sort of machine as the real foundation of the whole of an harmonious system, including many cells and many nuclei, because the development of this system goes on normally, even if its parts are rearranged or partly removed, and because a machine would never remain what it had been in such cases.[25]

Evidently for Driesch a material explanation such as Weismann's was a mechanical one. Moreover, the autonomy of vital phenomena of which Driesch spoke referred to the separation or independence of life from physical and chemical laws: "Life, at least morphogenesis, is not a specialised arrangement of inorganic events; biology, therefore, is not applied physics and chemistry: life is something apart, and biology is an independent science."[26] This autonomy of life could only be the work, on the other hand, of nonmaterial, nonmechanical agencies like Aristotle's formative and final causes, for Driesch believed he had shown in the regulative and regenerative capacity of the organism ". . . that there is at work a something in life phenomena 'which bears the end in itself'."[27]

The promulgation of the cell theory during the nineteenth century did more, however, than revive debate between vitalists and material preformationists of the Weismann school. It also provoked new discussions concerning the meaning of a "living being" or "organism." The plant and animal organisms with which biologists were familiar were now seen to be composed of smaller units, the cells, and these in turn were rapidly equated with previously observed microscopic forms of life, such as infusoria. Yet the latter were readily construed to be living beings, since they carried out all of the significant vital functions—assimilation of nutrients, growth, excretion, respiration, regulation, and reproduction—that the multicellular forms of life carried out as integrated assemblages of cells. The principal exponents of the cell theory recognized, therefore, that insofar as the cell contained the basic properties of life on which every organism depends, the cell became the ultimate term of analysis of living things. Theodor Schwann wrote of cells having an "independent life": "The cause of nutrition and growth resides not in the totality of the organism, but in its elementary parts, the cells."[28]

An interesting outcome of this view of life was that the multicellular organisms of the ordinary macroscopic world came to be regarded as collectivities. For Schwann the multicellular organism was a cellular state in which "each cell is a citizen."[29] Indeed, in such a cellular state there is a distribution of tasks, or division of labor. The whole depends upon the cooperation of the parts. This notion of the organism as collectivity was well put by Schleiden, who wrote as follows of plant cells: "Each cell leads a double life: an autonomous one with its own development, the other as an intermediary insofar as it has become an integrated part of the plant."[30]

On the one hand, therefore, entities considerably smaller than the macroscopic organisms of ordinary experience were recognized as organisms, even if they were only, to use Brücke's term, *elementary organisms*.[31] On the other hand, the metaphor of collectivity or social state that was increasingly applied to the multicellular organism probably revived older concepts of societies themselves as organisms. There was, in effect, little point in stopping at the level of the individual composed of spatially contiguous cells when conferring organismal status. The zoologist Alfred Espinas, for example, in reviewing the characteristics of various kinds of animal societies, discerned certain "laws" governing their behavior: the parts (individual organisms) of a society manifested a division of labor and relationships that were the outcome of epigenetic development and served to preserve the organized ensemble as a whole. In recognizing these fundamental properties of societies Espinas could not help but conclude that "societies were without doubt living beings [êtres vivants]."[32] Herbert Spencer was another prominent nineteenth-century figure to speak in a similar manner of "social organisms."[33]

If living beings could be discerned at higher levels of organization than had been previously considered, it was possible at least to imagine life at levels below that of the cell. Indeed, a century earlier the Count de Buffon had hypothesized the existence of *living organic molecules* which, when assimilated, accounted for the growth of organized beings, and which, when specifically arranged by the internal mold of these beings, accounted for their specific form. In some manner, not clearly defined by Buffon, the mold could reproduce and this property could eventuate in the formation of new organisms.[34] The nineteenth century witnessed a growing interest in such hypothetical invisible units that could, by the stroke of assigning them such vital properties as growth, reproduction, and variation, bid fair to resolve the difficulties of explaining the phenomenon of heredity. E. B. Wilson, in his classic *The Cell in Development and Inheritance*, catalogued fifteen versions of these hypothetical units, which included Spencer's *physiological units*, Darwin's *pangenes*, Nägeli's *micellae*, and Weismann's *biophores*.[35] While these hypothetical entities were useful in materialist theories, the lack of any empirical basis for their existence made them the susceptible target they proved to be in the contentious early years of the twentieth century.

III. Early Years of Genetics and Biochemistry

The vitalistic resurgence represented by Driesch's criticism of Weismann's theory may have had lingering effects on the evolution of the field of embryology during the twentieth century, but it soon aroused opposition in a corner of the biological sciences where two new fields, biochemistry and genetics, were emerging and rapidly converging. In 1897 the Buchner brothers had made the important discovery that the agent responsible for the acceleration of the alcoholic fermentation of sugar in yeast could be separated from the living cell.[36] Little fundamental differences could thereafter be recognized between the extracellular digestive enzymes secreted by cells and the "intracellular ferments": both were material substances capable of catalyzing chemical reactions responsible for significant activities of the cell. From the discovery of the Buchners' emerged a new field of biochemistry characterized by an increasing search for enzymes and their isolation from the cell. There also emerged a growing expectation, at least among biochemists, that the various activities of the cell could be attributed to the physicochemical properties of these isolated enzymes.[37] In 1900 the principles of Mendelian inheritance were reenunciated independently by DeVries, Correns, and Tschermak, this time with more resounding impact.[38] The existence of genetic factors, or genes, as the "determinants" of characters that arise in the course of development was given greater acceptance because of their value in predicting the quantitative outcome of "crosses" between individuals with contrasting hereditary characters. Among the champions of the new Mendelism was William Bateson, the English zoologist who coined the name of genetics for the new field and who was later to play an important role in making an early contact between genetics and biochemistry.

Influential at the turn of the century in relating the emerging fields of genetics and biochemistry was Jacques Loeb, who had emigrated nine years before from his native Germany to the United States. He saw in genes and enzymes a means of attacking a vitalistic conception of development. Indeed, he had behind him two experimental investigations that supported a viewpoint quite opposite to that of Driesch. The results of his work on heliotropisms in animals[39] indicated to him that behavior could be accounted for on a strictly physicochemical basis. Then his accomplishments in bringing about "artificial fertilization" (in reality, activation without sperm)[40] of sea urchin eggs by chemical procedures led him to suppose that the phenomenon of fertilization was as likely to have a physicochemical basis as was behavior. Interestingly enough, during his experiments on sea urchin embryos,[41] Loeb observed that immersion in diluted sea water would often cause a recently fertilized egg to extrude droplets of protoplasm. Upon becoming detached from the main mass of the egg, the droplet could eventually give rise to a "normal embryo." In drawing the conclusion that "every part of the protoplasm may give rise to fully developed embryos," Loeb must have realized he was veering dangerously close to Driesch's position that the egg was not a preorganized mechanism. Subsequently (1912), Loeb had to argue that a "prearrangement" or organization of "germ-regions" existed in the egg prior to fertilization, but that the separation of the different germ-regions did not occur until a later stage of development.[42]

Loeb's commitment to a mechanical, reductionist approach was made clear in an assessment of the "recent development in biology" which he wrote for *Science* in 1904:

... the investigations of the biologist differ from those of the chemist and physicist in that the biologist deals with the analysis of the mechanism of a special class of machines. Living organisms are chemical machines, made of essentially colloidal material which possess the peculiarity of developing, preserving and reproducing themselves automatically. The machines which have thus far been produced artificially lack the peculiarity of developing, growing, preserving and reproducing themselves, though no one can say with certainty that such machines might not one day be constructed artificially.[43]

Aware of the Buchners' discovery and of its significance for biology, Loeb wrote in the same article: "The progress made by chemistry, especially physical chemistry, had definitely put an end to the idea that the chemistry of living matter is different from the chemistry of inanimate matter. The presence of catalyzers in all living tissues makes it intelligible that in spite of the comparatively low temperature at which life phenomena occur the reaction velocities for the essential processes in living organisms are comparatively high."[44] In the same article Loeb also referred to the rediscovery of Mendelism and spoke of Mendel's paper as "one of the most prominent ever published in biology." He emphasized the quantitative, law-like statements and regarded them as auguring well for future studies of heredity.

Loeb had an opportunity to bring together these twin interests in biochemistry and genetics when he collaborated with W. O. R. King and A. R. Moore at the University of California in a study of hybridization between two Pacific Coast species of sea urchins, *Stronglyocentrotus purpuratus* and *S. franciscanus*.[45] The pluteus larvae of these two species differ in a number of characteristics: spininess of the skeleton, length of arms, cross bars in the skeleton, and body shape. By using the sperm of one species to fertilize the eggs of the other, Loeb and his collaborators found that not only could normal pluteus larvae be produced in this way, but the resulting hybrid larvae had largely the appearance of *franciscanus* larvae. Thus, the *franciscanus* characteristics appeared to exhibit Mendelian dominance.

These experiments became the basis of further investigations by A. R. Moore, then a graduate student, who made the careful observation that the *franciscanus* characters were only *partially* dominant, in that while these characters did emerge in the larvae eventually produced, the *rate* of their appearance was definitely slower in the hybrid.[46] For example, in the *franciscanus* larva cross bars grow out from lateral spines to meet in the midline. The rate at which this occurred was reduced in what Moore referred to as the "heterozygote," using the new genetic term originated by Bateson. Moore was in fact indebted to Bateson for more than a new language: In *Mendel's*

Principles of Heredity[47] Bateson developed his "presence and absence" hypothesis, according to which "the dominant character is due to the *presence* of something which in the case of the recessive is *absent.*"

Familiar with Garrod's studies on alcaptonuria,[48] Bateson made these remarks:

A correct knowledge of the system which a hereditary disease follows in the course of its descent will, it may be anticipated, contribute to a proper understanding of the pathology of these affections, and thus make a definite advance in the general study of the physiology of the disease. If, for example, a disease descends through the affected persons as a dominant, we may feel every confidence that the condition is caused by the operation of a factor or element added to the usual ingredients of the body: In such cases there is something *present*, probably a definite chemical substance,which has the power of producing the affection. . . . On the contrary, when the disease is recessive we recognize that its appearance is due to the *absence* of some ingredient which is present in the normal body. So, for example, albinism is almost certainly due to the absence of at least one of the factors, probably a ferment,[49] which is needed to cause the excretion of pigment; and, as Garrod has shown, alkaptonuria must be regarded as due to the absence of a certain ferment which has the power of decomposing the substance alkapton. In the normal body the substance is not present in the urine, because it has been broken up by the responsible ferment; but when the organism is deficient in the power to produce that ferment, then the alkapton is excreted undecomposed and the urine is colored by it.[50]

Indeed, Bateson went on to say, ". . . we may draw from Mendelian observations the conclusion that in at least a large group of cases the heredity of characters consists in the transmission of the power to produce something with properties resembling those of ferments. It is scarcely necessary to emphasise the fact that the ferment itself must not be declared to be the factor or thing transmitted, but rather, the power to produce that ferment, or ferment-like body."[51]

Given this idea and his observation of the retarded development of dominant characters in hybrid sea urchins, Moore proposed a biochemical explanation of incomplete or partial dominance.[52] He assumed each "unit-character" develops because a specific enzyme existed in the parental germ cell, and he accepted the Batesonian view that dominance is due to the presence of an enzyme and recessiveness to the absence of it. On these assumptions, an F_1 hybrid resulting from a cross between a dominant and a recessive must contain just half the amount of the enzyme found in the pure dominant. This followed from the fact that the heterozygote contained but one dose of the dominant factor,[53] whereas the pure dominant contained two doses. Moore was knowledgeable, too, about the effects of enzymes on reaction kinetics, as his mentor had recently reviewed the subject.[54] It was well known that when the concentration of substrate is large compared to the concentration of enzyme, reaction velocity is proportional to the concentration of enzyme. Moore indeed supposed that substrate was not limiting in the fertilized egg, but that in hybrids the concentration of enzyme limited the rate of reaction. In the course of time during development the amount of product (upon which the appearance of some character eventually depended) may approach in the hybrid that which is obtained in the pure dominant (since only the rate of reaction is affected, not the concentration of product at equilibrium). Therefore, hybrids may be expected to be more like the pure dominant with increasing time of development. He cited evidence to support this explanation in the case of the *Stronglyocentrotus* hybrids. He also pointed out that, if reactions are prevented from reaching equilibrium because of products of other reactions acting simultaneously (such as by consuming them chemically), then the hybrids may never get to look exactly like the pure dominants, and this would be the basis of incomplete or partial dominance.

In his 1912 paper Moore in fact referred to the work of Lang[55] on snails. In crosses of red with yellow snails, the heterozygous offspring when young were observed to be yellow, so that the ratio was initially 3 yellow to 1 red. However, as the heterozygotes grew older, they became red and the final ratio was 3 red: 1 yellow.

"The consequences of following the application of the laws of enzyme reactions have been discussed at length because evidence seems to point to the presence and action of enzymes in the phenomena of development [Moore argued]. . . . the inadequacy of the methods of the investigation which may have been used heretofore lies in attempting to measure only the end-products of the reactions and neglecting entirely the question of reaction velocity."[56]

Loeb was much taken with Moore's interesting interpretation of reduced developmental rate in heterozygotes as indicating hereditary control of enzyme amount. This approach provided additional support for Loeb's fundamental attitude of seeking explanation for vital phenomena in physicochemical processes. He had in the meantime been measuring the effect of the temperature on the rates of such biological processes as heart beat and egg cleavage. The extent to which a 10° change in temperature affected the rate had come to be called the Q_{10} of the process in question, and the value of the Q_{10} had come to indicate whether the process was a purely physical one or the result of chemical reactions. Q_{10}'s of 1 were taken as indicators of physical processes, whereas Q_{10}'s of 2 to 3 or higher were taken as indicators of chemically based processes.[57] Together with Ewald,[58] Loeb had shown that the heart beat of embryos of the fish *Fundulus* had a Q_{10} indicating that it was determined by the velocity of a chemical reaction. Moreover, they noted that at a given temperature all *Fundulus* embryos had practically the same heart beat. On the basis that, given a sufficient amount of substrate, the velocity of a chemical reaction in a living organism is proportional to the mass of enzyme catalyzing it, Loeb and Ewald concluded that all hearts of *Fundulus* embryos must contain the same mass of enzyme, since they all beat at the same rate when the temperature was the same. Loeb went further. Considering the rate of heart beat to be a hereditary character, he was ''forced to the conclusion that each embryo of *Fundulus* inherits practically the same mass of those enzymes which are responsible for the heart beat. The hereditary factor in this case must consist of material which determines the formation of a given mass of these enzymes, since the factors in the chromosomes are too small to carry the whole mass of the enzymes existing in the embryo or adult.''[59]

Despite the caution that Loeb here displayed in avoiding prematurely any identity between hereditary factor or gene, on the one hand, and enzyme on the other, the desire to identify the gene in chemical terms was revealed in a subsequent paper by Loeb and Chamberlain.[60] Their paper opened as follows: ''There is a general tendency to visualize the factors which determine the hereditary characters as specific chemical compounds. If we wish to carry this view (with which we sympathize) beyond the limit of a vague statement, we must either try to establish the nature of these compounds by the methods of the organic chemist, or we must use the methods of general or physical chemistry and try to find numerical relations by which we can identify the quantities of the reacting masses or the ratio in which they combine.''

It is unlikely that the tendency to view genes as specific chemical coumpounds was as widespread in 1915 as Loeb meant to imply. Surely Bateson could not be attributed as holding such a view;[61] nor was E. M. East, who had shown how quantitative characters in corn could be accounted for on the basis of many genes contributing to the same character, inclined to think of genes as more than convenient algebraic symbols.[62] In any event, despite the implied promise of the opening sentences, Loeb and Chamberlain offered little more in their paper than a plausible explanation for the differences they had observed in the rate of segmentation in different eggs of the sea-urchin *Arbacia*.[63]

Since the Q_{10} for the extent of variation of the rate of segmentation of the *Arbacia* egg was quite similar to the Q_{10} for the rate of segmentation itself, the variations could be readily accounted for as due to variation between different eggs in the mass of the segmentation enzymes they contained. Surely, it would have been foolhardy for Loeb and Chamberlain to conclude that different amounts of the hereditary factors responsible for segmentation were distributed between different eggs, and they refrained from doing so. The net result, however, was that the genetic factor remained chemically unidentified despite the quantitative data obtained in this case.

Yet the search for a relation between gene and enzyme continued to be pursued. Aware of the previously demonstrated role of tyrosin oxidation in the formation of melanin pigment, Huia Onslow, in England, tested extracts obtained from the coats of a variety of mammals for their power to produce black pigment from tyrosin *in vitro* in the presence of hydrogen peroxide. He found such a catalytic activity (later called tyrosinase) in the extracts obtained from darkly pigmented coats, but observed no such activity in extracts of coats of "self-yellow," a recessive variation.[64] Sewall Wright referred to this work when he published his important monograph on the genetic factors affecting coat color in guinea pigs.[65] Of these factors, four were interpreted, because of their very close linkage and their quantitative effect on the production of dark pigment, as "variations of the same thing" (what today we would refer to as "members of an allelic series"), as variations in "a factor which determines the power of producing tyrosinase." Wright was obviously careful to differentiate the power to produce an enzyme from the enzyme itself.

Nevertheless, in other quarters the desire to associate gene and enzyme in an intimate way was less thoroughly checked. In 1916 Richard Goldschmidt began reporting the results of extensive investigations, beginning in 1909, of different geographic races of the moth *Lymantria dispar*.[66] He reported that the result of hybridization between certain geographic races was a failure to obtain normal sexual dimorphism among the progeny: individuals of one sex assumed to a certain extent the characters of the other sex, that is, became intersexual. The degree of intersexuality was constant in a given cross, but it could vary in crosses between different races. The variations extended throughout the entire range of possibilities between maleness and femaleness, the extremes being complete transformation of females into males, or vice versa, so that only one sex might be found among the offspring of a particular interracial cross. Such a transformation occurred not only in regard to the primary sexual characters of gonadal type and structure of genitalia but also in regard to secondary sexual characters, such as pigmentation of the wing scales, which is different in the two sexes. When a cross resulted in intersexual offspring, the reciprocal cross was normal. In the second (F_2) generation from crosses yielding intersexual offspring, intersexuality was found to segregate and there were definite patterns of transmission of male and female intersexuality.

Goldschmidt was able to account for all of these results by supposing that in *Lymantria* individuals of each sex contained "genetic factors" for both sexes. Which sexual characteristics were expressed depended upon the quantitative relation between the two sets of factors. Transmission of the male-determining factors was best accounted for by supposing they were carried by the chromosomes, whereas female-determining factors (F) were in the cytoplasm. In an ordinary intraracial cross, males and females were segregated among the offspring in equal proportions because, while each sex contained the same female-determining factors in the cytoplasm, males were homozygous for a chromosomal gene M, whereas females were heterozygous (Mm) having one allele (m) less potent as a male determiner than the other (M). Nevertheless, the determination of sex could be regarded as the outcome of a competition between the male- and female-determining factors, both of which influenced the same characters but in different directions. In an intraracial cross, the potencies of the two types of sex factors were so balanced that femaleness was assured in heterozygotes (MmF), maleness in homozygotes (MMF). The potencies of M and F were assumed to differ considerably in different races, so that in an interracial cross the M factors of one race might be insufficient, for example, to overcome the F factor of the other (or conversely) so as to produce intersexes in the hybrids.

Goldschmidt saw in these results not only a special mechanism of sexual differentiation, different from the XX–XY mechanism already observed in other animals, but also persuasive evidence of a catalytic effect of the gene in the physiological processes of development. In his brief note in *Science* in 1916, Goldschmidt argued that from an inspection of the wings of a graded series of intersexes one could infer "immediately that there must be an amount of pigment, or more correctly, of oxidase [tyrosinase] quantitatively fixed, and corresponding to the quantitative value of m–f [difference between the potencies of the male and female-determining factors of the organism]; and that the given quantity (or concentration) flows out from the veins over the scales, wherever it happens to come." Thus, Goldschmidt claimed to have demonstrated that "a quantitative difference in the potency of hereditary factors causes a parallel, quantitatively different enzyme production."

In "A further contribution to the theory of sex" published in 1917,[67] Goldschmidt elaborated on the results he had been obtaining in interracial hybridization of *Lymantria* as well as upon the usefulness of his hypothesis to account for the facts. Goldschmidt began with an assumption, similar to A. T. Moore's, that the rate of development depends upon the potency of enzymes, which is the result of their concentration and activity. So far as sex determination in *Lymantria* was concerned, however, both male- and female-determining enzymes were hypothesized to be present in both sexes. On this hypothesis, therefore, the sex outcome is determined by which set of enzymes was more potent, simply because the differentiation of an organ occurs at a given time during development. If the male-determined enzyme, for example, has been more rapidly building up specific determining substances than has the female-determining enzyme, that organ will become male-like and complete its differentiation before products of the female-determining enzyme become effective. Intersexes come to be explained on this basis in an obvious way: in intersexes, enzymes of both sexes produce products at rates sufficient to make both effective at around the same time, so that an organ affected by both enzymes develops along both male and female pathways at the same time.

This preoccupation with enzymes as causative agents of organ differentiation during development brought Goldschmidt to his next explanatory leap. How were the genetically determined differences in enzymatic potency to be accounted for? He might have argued that hereditary factors governed the potencies of enzymes in some as yet inexplicable way. But he proposed instead a simpler solution: the genetic factors of genes were the enzymes themselves. In the opening of his 1917 paper, Goldschmidt stated:

When we use Mendelian formulae we are expressing the fact that unknown things, for which the Mendelian symbols stand, behave as units in inheritance and are distributed among the offspring of an organism unchanged and according to definite laws. When we talk about sex-factors, therefore, we only express the view that the sexual differences are due to different combinations of things of the same type as those which stand for genetic differences of other kinds, things which we symbolize as unit-factors. . . . And now the question arises whether the results of our experiments do not enable us to replace our symbolistic interpretation by a physiological one.[68]

Later in the paper, after demonstrating the relation between the combination of sex factors and rate of developmental processes, he asserted: "From these facts only one conclusion can at present be drawn: that the sex-factors are enzymes (or bodies with the properties of enzymes) which accelerate a reaction according to their concentration."[69]

In brief, like Loeb and Chamberlain, Goldschmidt believed it desirable to identify the gene in chemical terms, but was less hesitant than they in concluding that the genes were enzymes, because enzymatically catalyzed reactions were affected by genes. Today we recognize the conclusion to be in error, but Goldschmidt's rapid jump in the interpretation of experimental results is cited here merely to emphasize the early desire to link hereditary factor and physiological catalyst.

IV. Troland's Theories of Autocatalysis and Heterocatalysis

It would be a mistake to suggest that all investigators of heredity and development in the early years of the twentieth century were in agreement about this connection between gene and physiological process. In fact, the views of an early dissenter are particularly instructive. In a paper[70] delivered in January 1909 before the Biological Club at the University of Chicago, Oscar Riddle revealed his doubts about the validity of invoking Mendelian "factors" to account for patterns of heredity. His doubts were based, however, upon an assumption, not yet shown to be erroneous, that the hereditary factors were obligatorily involved in the biochemical activities of the cells to which they were transmitted. In his paper he drew upon evidence already obtained by others in studying abnormal tyrosine metabolism and pathological melanin pigmentations in the mammalian body. This evidence, he pointed out, served "to illustrate the dependence of tyrosin oxidations upon somatic conditions which may be of such a temporary, intermittent, quantitative or reversible character as to preclude the possibility of accounting for them on the basis of specific, independent transmissions, once for all segregated by the germ cells."[71]

Riddle referred, for example, to the case of melanotic tumors in otherwise albino horses. Obviously, in this case melanin production is not prevented permanently in these genetic albinos, for in tumorous growths of these animals melanin formation can occur. Similarly, citing work on the color of amphibian integuments, Riddle pointed out that, at various times between the larval and adult stage, pigmentation could be determined at will by controlling the physiological state, particularly the nutrition, of the animals. From both of these cases, one may conclude, as he apparently did, that the capacity for melanin formation could be present without being realized. But it is entirely possible, as our modern conception would have it, that the material genetic factor underlying this capacity may be present and even transmitted without being expressed. Riddle himself failed to recognize this alternative view which keeps the transmission of genetic factors distinct from their mode of action in the physiology of development. Rather, he was prepared to give up the concept of Mendelian genes. In a cross involving alternative characters (such as pigmented vs. albino), Riddle proposed that "it is the *power to oxidize tyrosine* compounds (a power which I believe, by no stretch of the imagination, needs to be or can be, represented by a particle in the germ, but by a general property of the protoplasm of germ cells and of tissue cells) *that is transmitted* and that here this power of *one* of the gametes is *continued into* the zygote without being very *appreciably* increased or diminished" (italics are Riddle's.)[72]

On this basis, of course, it is difficult to comprehend how such a general property or power is segregated the way it is in a cross. Riddle admitted this problem in saying: "How then on my view of the basis of color inheritance may the segregation and proportions which result in Mendelian behavior be accounted for? I must say at once that I do not know; but in this respect I consider myself hardly worse off than the wisest Mendelian. My supposition, however, would put less faith than theirs in the behavior of chromosomes during the maturation divisions."[73] He simply supposed that in certain organisms maturation division somehow resulted regularly in one gamete with a high potency to oxidize melanin for every one with a low potency.

Riddle's objections were raised in 1909. By 1915, when *The Mechanism of Mendelian Heredity* was published,[74] the evidence had become much more impressive that genes were material entities. In brief, Morgan's school had shown that genes were transmitted in linearly arranged groups, which were equal in number to the number of chromosomes in the gametes, and that an abnormal transmission of a chromosome, as visually detected in cytological studies, was reflected in a correspondingly abnormal transmission of a gene, as detected in the outcome of a breeding experiment. If, then, genes owed their properties of transmission and segregation to their physical residence on chromosomes, to what did they owe their powers of affecting the outcome of developmental processes? Would it be possible to reconcile, within the context of a material hereditary factor, the properties of transmission and potency in developmental determination? The most important attempt to offer such a reconciliation was that of Leonard Thompson Troland, then completing his graduate studies at Harvard University.[75] Troland brought to this problem an extensive knowledge of the electrical properties of what were at the time called the colloidal particles of the cell.[76] He was particularly interested in the possibility of accounting for enzymatic catalysis in terms of the then accepted notions of colloidal surface structure. His knowledge of the three-dimensional structure of what today we recognize as macromolecules was obviously primitive from a modern viewpoint, but the intellectually seminal importance of Troland's work lay in his sensing a connection between catalysis, on the one hand, and the twin properties of the hereditary material, transmission and developmental intervention, on the other.

Troland had, in fact, seized upon recently enunciated ideas, stemming from Loeb's early emphasis upon catalysts in vital phenomena, that the autocatalytic formation of a crystal was analogous to that of biological growth and gene reproduction.[77] But the reasons for his interest in the problem of relating catalysis to hereditary properties went further. An early version of his so-called "enzyme theory of life" was presented in 1914 in a philosophical journal, *The Monist*. Entitled "The chemical origin and regulation of life,"[78] this paper had as its avowed purpose the combatting of the thesis of the "new vitalism" displayed in the works of Driesch in Germany and Henri Bergson[79] in France. Troland, like Loeb, was averse to vitalistic views. Recognizing that the regulative capacity of life was the property that vitalists believed to require invocation of extra-physical explanations, he sought a way of accounting for regulation in material terms. He realized that "Regulation is essentially a selective capacity. Out of a multitude of possible chemical and physical reactions the living organism selects only those limited few which correspond to what we call its 'needs' and 'purposes.'"[80] It appeared to him that all vital activity involved chemical change, which observation led him to look for, "a material principle of regulation having an essentially chemical nature and function." To Troland the enzyme was the principle par excellence. "The enzyme," he wrote, "is an organic catalyst, and a catalyst is a substance which by its mere presence in a mixture is able to facilitate and direct the chemical changes there taking place. This directive power of a catalyst resides wholly in its singular ability to accelerate the so-called reaction velocity of specific chemical reactions.[81] Moreover, very little enzyme was necessary to effect a great deal of chemical change, as the enzyme was unconsumed in the process.

Troland pointed out that the manner in which the catalyst did this was still unknown, but he felt certain that "modern electrical theory of the constitution of matter" would provide a simple explanation, one that would be in harmony with all existing physical and chemical principles. The important considera- tion was that specific catalyzers, or enzymes, were found in protoplasm. These enzymes essentially increased the rate of chemical change in living organisms to such a degree that activity seemed to occur where otherwise it would not. With this knowledge of the enzyme's power, Troland found it possible to resolve what he called the five fundamental mysteries of vital behavior: (1) the origin of living matter, (2) the origin of organic variations, (3) the ground of heredity, (4) the mechanism of individual development, and (5) the basis of physiological regulation in the mature organism.

So far as the creation of life was concerned, Troland invited his readers to imagine that a small amount of "enzyme" appeared at some point in the Paleozoic ocean. The "enzyme" had the capacity to increase the rate of formation of some oily substance immiscible with water; the oil droplet grew as a consequence of enzymatic action and eventually broke up into a number of smaller globules. These globules receiving no "enzyme" would have been unable to continue the process further, and so for continued reproduction an enzyme must have appeared having the *additional* power of autocatalysis. Besides having the power to aid in the formation of substances unlike itself, the autocatalytic "enzyme" was also able to aid in the formation of more "enzyme." "It is only necessary," he theorized, "that the enzyme about which [the globule] centers should be autocatalytic, as well as effective in the production of primitive protoplasm. In this case each new globule which is formed from the original one may carry away with it a quantity of enzyme sufficient to permit its continuous growth and reproduction."[82]

So far as the source of the original enzyme was concerned, Troland admit- ted that it would have to have been a very improbable event in the Paleozoic ocean, the outcome of some fortuitous collision of atoms and molecules. Nevertheless, the improbable is not impossible. Once such an "enzyme" appeared with autocatalytic powers, life may be said to have begun: "That control of self and environment, which the vitalist rightly regards as [life's] defining feature, appertains to life only by virtue of the store of *enzymes* which is hidden away in the protoplasm, and when one of these enzymes first appeared, bare of all body, in the aboriginal seas it followed as a consequence of its characteristic regulative nature that the phenomena of life came too."[83] Troland assured his philosophical readers that there was nothing mysterious about autocatalysis, that it had been observed in the field of inorganic chemistry (although no examples were given in this work) and so was not a vitalistic phenomenon.

Troland admitted that the original droplets of "primitive protoplasm" were, because of their homogeneity, probably unlike the heterogenous, complex protoplasm we know today. But "modern" protoplasm could have been the result of a chemical history, an evolutionary process depending upon the occurrence of variations in the autocatalytic "enzyme" itself. For endowment with autocatalytic powers does not "preclude the occurrence of further chance events of the same general kind as the one which produced the first 'enzyme'; indeed, on account of the increase in chemical activity which it occasions the presence of the catalyzer decidedly favors such further events."[84] This means that, if enough time elapsed, a second autocatalytic "enzyme" would arise by chance variation from the first. Most of these variations would be unlikely to facilitate reactions favorable to their continued existence and thus would be destroyed. But if a variation did arise that facilitated such reactions, it would be preserved by the action of natural selection. In this way Troland's "enzyme theory of life," as he called it, provided "a molecular basis for organic variation." Indeed, a new "enzyme" arising by random variation might have become part of a more complex germ plasm if it added to rather than replaced some of the original unchanged ones. "In this way, as time goes on, the organic forms which exist upon the earth will tend to become more and more complex."[85]

The remaining mysteries of life seemed to be elucidated quite readily, once these basic tenets of the "enzyme theory of life" were accepted. The "ground of heredity" was the set of "native ferments" contained in the nucleus of the germ cell.

". . . . the cell nucleus is supposed in the theory of Weismann to contain the hereditary determinants, and hence, in our hypothesis, the enzymes."[86]

Since only a very small amount of catalytic substance was necessary for catalysis, a germ cell could contain lots of enzymatic material sufficient to contain representatives of the enzymes of all parts of the body. Following fertilization, these "enzymes" were sorted out during the mitotic divisions that segment the fertilized ovum into numerous cells. Certain cells retained the full battery of "enzymes" contained in the nucleus of the fertilized ovum. These cells were the future germ cells, as well as "latent cells" lodged within the various kinds of somatic tissue that received only parts of the germinal complement of "enzymes." The somatic cells that were deprived of some set of germinal "enzymes" were thereby differentiated, in line with Weismann's theory. Having a full complement of enzymatic material, the "latent cells" left behind among the somatic cells were capable of regenerating any required 'lost part', given the appropriate stimulus. Thus, the "latent cells" could explain the phenomena of regulation and regeneration that Driesch found refractory to mechanistic interpretation. Finally, the fact that the chemical changes occurring in the mature organism "are almost invariably of the right kind, and occur in the right place" was itself the consequence of the original enzymatic material in the germ. Thus, the seemingly teleological regulation of chemical reactions in the organism was again accounted for by the capacity of the "enzymes" in the soma and "latent cells" to direct specific chemical reactions, and this directive or regulative capacity was the outcome of natural selection.

In short, the "enzyme theory of life" as propounded in the *Monist* article was regarded by Troland as a successful "rebuttal of vitalism," inasmuch as "enzymes" could be shown to be involved in the creation of life, to be the basis of evolution and of the development, differentiation, and regulative functioning of organisms. The "enzyme," in Troland's words, replaced Driesch's entelechy as "the pilot of life's journey." The term "enzyme" was used by him, as we have seen, as synonymous with a particular kind of biological *catalyst*, a molecule capable of both autocatalytic and heterocatalytic activity. This catalyst was not necessarily supposed to be a protein, although it was believed to reside primarily in the nucleus and secondarily in the cytoplasm. The stress, then, was upon catalysis rather than any specific class of organic molecules.

These views of Troland, originally presented in fairly general form for a philosophical audience, were strengthened and fleshed out with scientific detail in a subsequent paper designed for biologists, the next group of individuals to be protected against the incursions of vitalism. This paper, "Biological Enigmas and the Theory of Enzyme Action," was published in 1917 in the *American Naturalist*,[87] which at that time enjoyed an extremely wide readership among biologists. Geneticists and evolutionary biologists, in particular, contributed to and read the influential theoretical and experimental papers published in that journal. Troland's motives were overt. He wished to chastise biologists for their recent return to vitalism and their failure to see in the rapidly developing physical sciences the basis for ultimate explanations of the fundamental biological enigmas. In particular, he would have biologists see in specific catalysis a solution for all the "fundamental biological enigmas." After all, "catalysis is essentially a *determinative* relationship. . . ." (italics mine), and his conception of life "would claim that all intra-vital or 'hereditary' determination is, in the last analysis, catalytic." Indeed, this conception "links these great biological phenomena [heredity, evolution, ontogeny and general organic regulation] directly with molecular physics and perfects the unity not alone of biology, but of the whole system of physical science, by suggesting that what we call life is fundamentally a product of catalytic laws acting in colloidal systems of matter throughout the long periods of geologic time."[88]

What were these catalytic laws on which Troland placed so much weight? He drew upon the available knowledge of catalysis and crystal structure,[89] indulging in the speculation that there might be no fundamental difference between crystalloids (what we today would call small molecules) and colloids (today's marcromolecules). Colloidal particles of starch or protein were held to be polymeric in the sense that they had a lattice structure, with molecules at repeated distances, like that of a crystal, and were not thought of as being macromolecular in the sense of having periodic, covalently bonded monomeric units. Thinking in these terms, he accepted the analogy of catalysis as crystal formation, supposing the former to consist in the deposition or adsorption of reacting substances upon the surfaces of colloidal particles, like the deposition of molecules of a given species upon an already existing crystal lattice of such molecules.

Troland stressed the distinction, however, between two types of catalysis: *autocatalysis,* or the change in velocity of a reaction generating more of the catalyst; and *heterocatalysis,* or change in the velocity of a reaction altering the structure of a different substance. Autocatalysis was illustrated by crystallization in a supersaturated solution. The physical description of the formation of a crystal would account for the "synthesis of polymeric molecules from individual units which are all alike." If a crystal surface consisted "of an orderly arrangement of. . . . two molecular groupings in mosaic or lattice form," it would attract in the same way the molecules of the solute and "the crystal or polymeric molecule would be built up out of two components by the simultaneous and parallel action of two initially combined species of molecular fields."[90] The change was catalyzed by the crystal and was an autocatalytic process involving the joining (apparently without covalent linkage) of two substances. Such an explanation could, of course, be expanded to cover the case of a polymeric molecule made up of several different kinds of component molecules. "The catalytic surface thus acts like an orienting sieve which on account of its special structure forces a chaotic crowd of individuals which come into contact with it, to fall into a special configuration."[91] However, unlike crystallization, "the products of catalysis do not adhere permanently to the catalytic surface." When the field of force weakens as the polymeric molecules grow, a portion of it detaches. Thus, the making of separate duplicate structures is achieved.

For Troland, heterocatalysis was regarded "as an extension of the process of autocatalysis." Exact similarity of the force patterns of the catalyzing and catalyzed systems was not essential in this case. Indeed, the catalytic effect was probably stronger when there was a complementary structural correspondence such as between a body and its mirror-image, or to use Emil Fischer's phrase, between a lock and its key. The catalytic surface probably exerted three influences: first, a local increase in the concentration of reacting substances at the surface; second, impressment upon the attached molecules of a relative orientation favorable to chemical union; and third, a weakening of the fields of force of the molecules due to their interaction with the surface fields. Thus, the catalyst increased the probability of effective collisions over that occurring by chance in the absence of the catalyst.

Troland's theory was hardly original, leaning as heavily as it did upon the already suggested analogy between catalysis and crystal formation. Nor did the theory enjoy much in the way of direct support, although the plausibility of the analogy lent it some physicochemical solidity. The main point was that one could readily conceive of a material entity having at once autocatalytic and heterocatalytic properties. Once accepting the possibility of such entities, the biological consequences were obvious, and Troland spelled them out for the biologist. The consequences were those he had already described in his *Monist* paper: these catalytic particles could grow and reproduce; they could specify chemical reactions in their immediate environment, and by undergoing occasional variations in structure they could evolve. Troland was very much aware of Mendelism and of the demonstration by Morgan's school of the existence of Mendelian factors on chromosomes.[92] All one had to do, therefore, was to suppose that such catalytic particles made up the chromatin substance of the nucleus, and the demonstrable properties of the hereditary material in the chromosomes were accounted for in physicochemical terms:

"Although the fundamental life property of the chromatin units is that of autocatalysis, it is necessary and legitimate to suppose that the majority of them sustain specific heterocatalytic relationships to reactions occurring in living matter."[93] Thus, the connection between heredity and development was explained. Since Mendelian factors in the chromosomes had been shown to determine the distinctive properties of cells, tissues, and species, and since these properties had been shown by Loeb, Moore, and Goldschmidt to be the result of the actions of enzymes, Troland assumed that the hereditary factors, his auto-heterocatalytic particles, were "enzymes." He knew of Bateson's caution that the genetic factors might only be responsible for the production of enzymes, but he felt that in the absence of any evidence inconsistent with this assumption, it was simplest to equate "genetic factors" and "enzymes." In the relatively undeveloped state of chemical knowledge about the cell nucleus, it was too early to say much about the chemical nature of these "genetic factors," but Troland hazarded the guess that they might prove to be nucleic acids, since these substances appeared to be "the permanent and essential component of the nucleus." Moreover, he added prophetically; "If, as now seems probable, the genetic enzymes must be identified with the nucleic acids, we shall be forced to suppose that these substances, although homogeneous—in animal or plant—from the point of view of ordinary chemical analysis, are actually built up in the living chromatin, into highly differentiated colloidal, and colloidal-molar structures."[94]

The chemical identification of the "genetic enzymes" was in any case, for Troland, secondary to more compelling biological issues. He was intent upon showing how his "enzyme theory"—a theory of autocatalytic particles with heterocatalytic properties—vitiated the force of Driesch's argument that to explain the reproduction of a nuclear "machine" one must postulate another machine to carry out the operation, and so on *ad infinitum*. Troland's "enzymes" could intervene in development because of their heterocatalytic functions, but they could reproduce as well, needing no outside "machine" to accomplish this function. Moreover, by the time of his *American Naturalist* paper, he was able to free himself from a purely Weismannian scheme of development. He realized that he no longer needed "latent" cells to account for the regulative capacity of the embryo. The "enzyme theory" made unnecessary Weismann's argument that embryological development resulted from differential segregation of genetic determinants. Rudimentary differentiation could result from environmental differences acting on a group of cells that were otherwise alike in their content of genetic factors. Environmental differences between cells could ensue from their different positions in the embryonic mass, for example. In different environments the heterocatalytic activities of the genetic factors might differ without necessarily affecting their power to reproduce. In so disjoining the autocatalytic from the heterocatalytic function of the genetic factor, Troland was making possible a clear realization that the hereditary material could be transmitted without being expressed in some line of cells arising in the course of development.

Finally, Troland wanted his biologist-reader to see that his autocatalytic particles with heterocatalytic functions had the very properties of life. They lent themselves to evolution because variant forms of these particles might arise through fortuitous collisions with the appropriate molecules. These new particles, or mutations, would be removed by natural selection if they failed to preserve the organism, either by failing in their autocatalytic function or by executing their heterocatalytic function in an inefficient way. On the other hand, if the autocatalytic or heterocatalytic function were rendered more efficient by mutation, the mutant form would in fact enjoy a selective advantage. Finally, if one traced evolution far enough back in time, one must come to the "first mutation," that is, the molecular production of an autocatalytic particle sustaining relations with its environment so as to make possible its continued growth and reproduction. That was in reality the origin of life. The simplest typical life structure would therefore be a free autocatalytic particle surrounded by an envelope of semiliquid and a chemically homogeneous substance with which it sustained a heterocatalytic relationship. From such a simple organism evolution could lead, through complexity in composition and consequent complexity of heterocatalytic activity, to more sophisticated "organisms" and eventually to the kinds of organisms we witness today.

V. The Gene as Organism

Troland did not retreat from the consequences of his theory. He knew that he was essentially regarding his hereditary catalysts as elementary organisms and that such conclusions might meet with strong opposition from such biologists as C. M. Child, a famous developmental biologist and member of the same department as Oscar Riddle at the University of Chicago. In his book, *Senescence and Rejuvenation,* [95] published in 1915, Child opposed any notion of hereditary particles for reasons somewhat different from those of Riddle. Child apparently saw in the kinds of hypothetical entities that E. B. Wilson had catalogued the common objectionable feature of being assigned the very properties they were invented to explain. In referring to corpuscular theories of the genetic material, Child wrote,

> The hypothetical units are themselves organisms with all the essential characteristics of the organisms that we know; they possess a definite constitution, they grow at the expense of nutritive material, they reproduce their kind. In other words, the problems of development, growth and reproduction, and inheritance exist for each of them, and the assumption of their existence brings us not a step nearer the solution of any of these problems. . . . No valid evidence for the existence of these units exists, but if their existence were to be demonstrated we might well despair of gaining any actual knowledge of life. [96]

In his *American Naturalist* article, Troland mentioned this argument only to rebut it. In the first place, Child appeared to have underestimated the importance of the facts already arrayed by geneticists pointing to a corpuscular determination of organismic activities. In short, the evidence for the existence of hereditary particles was at hand. [97] Second, Child's fear of attributing the vital properties of growth, development, and reproduction to the particles themselves was unfounded, since, as Troland had shown, the properties resided in the autocatalytic and heterocatalytic potential of certain substances. In fact, Troland was sure that autocatalytic activity was a property of all chemical substances, ". . . given the appropriate chemical environment. Since the environment of the chromatin particles has been made to order by evolution, the force of Child's criticims would seem to be nil." [98]

In brief, Troland saw no escape from accepting "enzymes" as elementary organisms, although he preferred his own term over such terms as "biophors"

(Weismann's term) or "determinants" or "factors," since these latter terms lacked a physical model or reference. The significant point was that Troland regarded these elementary organisms, rather than cells, as the ultimate explanatory units in biology.

Biologists who were less eager than Troland to consider the Mendelian factors, or genes, as elementary organisms could accept the distinction between genotype and phenotype that Johannsen had proposed,[99] without accepting any particular physicochemical model for it. In a real sense the genotype-phenotype distinction of Johanssen paralled Troland's distinction between autocatalysis and heterocatalysis; the genotype referred to that which is stably transmitted in heredity, while the phenotype referred to the development of characters in which the genotype participated. Yet the notion of a genotype does not presuppose any material basis for the recognized stability and regularity inherent in heredity. Indeed, Johannsen himself was impatient with attempts to materialize the genotype and equate genes with self-replicating units.[100] Thomas Hunt Morgan was only slightly less conservative. In his 1917 paper on "The Theory of the Gene," Morgan argued that while the concept of the gene as a discrete entity was *necessary* to explain the rules of hereditary transmission, there was a common misunderstanding arising from "a confusion of the problems concerned with sorting out of the hereditary materials, (the genes) to the eggs and sperms, with the problems concerning the subsequent action of these genes in the development of the embryo."[101]

In short, the distribution of genes in heredity told us nothing about the action of genes during embryonic development, and Morgan therefore argued "the importance of keeping apart, *for the present at least* [italics are Morgan's], the questions connected with the distribution of genes in succeeding generations from questions connected with the physiological action of the genetic factors during development."[102] Morgan wished to preserve the concept of the gene without pressing too hard about its physical nature, particularly as adduced from its presumed action in development.

H. J. Muller, on the other hand, appreciated early the significance of Troland's theoretical contribution. Muller had collaborated with T. H. Morgan, C. B. Bridges, and A. H. Sturtevant in establishing the linear arrangement of the genes in the visible chromosomes of the nucleus, thereby emphasizing the material reality of genes. Moreover, for some time before Troland's publications, he had been struck with the autocatalytic capability of chromatin, as evidenced in the notes he prepared in 1912 for an unpublished work on "Principles of Heredity."[103] It was not until 1921, when Muller delivered his paper on "Variation Due to Change in the Individual Gene" before the American Society of Naturalists, that he could do full justice to this theme. In that paper Muller made two cautions about Troland's theory and stressed one particular property of the gene. He pointed out that the specific metabolic enzymes whose activity depended upon the presence of certain genes should properly be regarded as phenotypic characters, and that the gene should no more be identified with enzymes than with any other character of the organism dependent upon gene expression. In short, to use Troland's terms, enzymes might themselves be the product of the gene's heterocatalytic function. The other caution was that Troland's analogy of gene duplication with crystal formation might prove to be inaccurate. Yet there was some merit to this notion of auto-attraction (attraction between portions of a molecule and similar building-blocks), for it could not only account for gene synthesis but also for the cytologically observed phenomenon of synapsis of homologous chromosomes. The matter to be emphasized was autocatalysis:

The most distinctive characteristic of each of these ultra microscopic particles—that characteristic whereby we identify it as a gene—is its property of self-propagation: the fact that, within the complicated environment of the cell protoplasm, it reacts in such a way as to convert some of the common surrounding material into an end-product identical in kind with the original gene itself. This action fulfills the chemist's definition of 'autocatalysis'; it is what the physiologist would call "growth"; and when it passes through more than one generation it becomes "heredity".... But the most remarkable feature of the situation.... is the fact that, when the structure of the gene becomes changed, through some "chance variation," the catalytic property of the gene may become correspondingly changed, in such a way as to leave it still autocatalytic.... for it is not inheritance *and* variation which brings about evolution, but the inheritance *of* variation, and this in turn is due to the general principle of gene construction which causes the persistence of autocatalysis despite the alteration in structure of the gene itself. Given, now, any material or collection of materials having this one unusual characteristic, and evolution would automatically follow."[104]

Muller's 1921 paper was interesting, too, for other reasons. He gave a hint there of his future course of work, the induction of mutations, for which he was later to receive the Nobel Prize. If the gene is a material entity capable of undergoing spontaneous mutation, he argued, it ought to be possible to alter environmental conditions so as to increase the rate of mutation: ". . . mutation is not a sacred, inviolable, unapproachable process: it may be altered."[105]

Muller also referred in this paper to the discovery of bacterial viruses, which had the same properties of propagability and mutation as did genes. This was hardly likely to be a coincidence and, since viruses were small and purifiable and capable of being studied in a test tube, he was induced to make his famous prediction "that perhaps we may be able to grind genes in a mortar and cook them in a beaker after all."[106] This was a clear, clarion call to move from treating genes exclusively as abstract units useful to account for the results of breeding experiments toward treating them as chemical entities with discoverable structure and properties.

In 1926 Muller returned to another theme broached by Troland. This was the theme of gene as organism, as the basis of life. In 1926 Muller gave an address in Ithaca, New York, before the International Congress of Plant Sciences in a symposium on "The Gene." The paper was long and covered much of what was then known about the size and number of genes and their arrangement in chromosomes. A final section was devoted, however, to the questions: "Could there ever have been a time, in the evolution of living matter, prior to the existence of what we may permissibly term the genes, and, at or before the time when genes did arise, how complicated could living matter have been, and what could have been its properties?"[107]

There followed an interesting argument ending in a conclusion quite similar to one earlier arrived at by Troland, that "life" did not occur before the gene. Muller's argument may be stated here in simplified form: "Living" involves growth, and growth involves autocatalysis. But autocatalysis in living matter is special; it is specific: those particular reactions are caused to occur whereby the autocatalyst is produced. Moreover, the autocatalyst is mutable, that is, can change in structure so as to have new (heterocatalytic) effects upon its substrate without losing the power of propagation. But

... it is almost inconceivable that a whole system of substances as that which any protoplasm or cytoplasm is conceived to be, should have come together by the chance action of physical and chemical substances, to form just such a structure that the working of this system reproduced the same system again, in all its features—*unless* the whole mechanism of biological evolution, including reproduction, variations, the reproduction of variations, and natural selection, had long previously been at work building up this system in just the right way from much simpler beginnings, that is, unless substances that may, in effect, be called genes existed first.[108]

From a simple autocatalytic agent, by definition a gene (even if not identical with any "modern" gene), our present-day protoplasm must have arisen, therefore, gradually, step by step, as successive mutations and natural selection resulted in a more complex "protoplasm" surrounding the genic material.

By 1947, when Muller wrote the Pilgrim Trust Lecture on "The Gene,"[109] he had further refined his thinking on all of these themes. By 1947, too, the possibility that nucleic acid might be the stuff of which genes were made had to be seriously considered,[110] and so the simple notion that the cell's enzymes, known to be proteins, were also the genes had to be held in abeyance, if not discarded. Moreover, the structure of a polymeric macromolecule was better understood as that of a covalently bonded chain of different building-blocks, allowing for variant arrangements.[111] Autocatalysis itself had been shown to occur in a variety of ways, some trivial with respect to the possible mechanism of gene reproduction. With respect to autocatalysis, for example, pepsin had been found to catalyze its own formation by digesting away a portion of a similar precursor molecule, pepsinogen.[112] This was unlikely to be the way genes were synthesized. The distinctive feature of gene reproduction, Muller noted, was that "complicated chemical changes are induced by the self-duplicating agent that could not take place otherwise, and that from a heterogeneous medium which may be alike for many different agents and in this sense non-specific, the agent selects the components necessary for itself and arranges and combines them into a form modelled on its own."[113] This was not a common property of matter, contrary to what Troland implied in referring to autocatalysis as universally potential in matter. For this reason, "autocatalytic" and "heterocatalytic" were changed, in the hope of preventing confusion, to "autosynthetic" and "heterosynthetic." Yet the principal distinction of Troland's remained—the former referred to the construction of a new gene based on the model of the old, while the latter referred to synthesis of materials different from the gene itself.

Following Muller's early espousal of the idea of gene as autocatalyst, the concept took hold of several other influential geneticists. J. B. S. Haldane, in an essay on "The Origin of Life" written in 1928,[114] referred, for example, to Muller's perceptive comparison of a bacterial virus to a gene. Recognizing that both require a rich organic environment in order to reproduce, Haldane went on to speculate about the possible origin of life. He imagined an early time in the history of the planet earth when the atmosphere contained little or no oxygen, when ultraviolet light could therefore penetrate easily to the earth's surface (lacking an ozone layer to impede the radiation), and when organic materials could gradually be built up through the action of ultraviolet light on water, carbon dioxide, and ammonia. Neither oxygen nor forms of life were yet present to prevent the accumulation of a vast array of complex macromolecules.

The first living or half-living things were probably large molecules synthesized under the influence of the sun's radiation, and only capable of reproduction in the particularly favorable medium in which they originated. Each presumably required a variety of highly specialized molecules before it could reproduce itself, and it depended on chance for a supply of them. This is the case today with most viruses, including the bacteriophage [bacterial virus], which can grow only in the presence of the complicated assortment of molecules found in a living cell.[115]

The similarity of these views to those of Troland is, of course, obvious, as are the following views concerning the mode of gene reproduction:

The growth and reproduction of large molecules are not, it may be remarked, quite hypothetical processes. They occur, it would seem, in certain polymerizations which are familiar to organic chemists. In my opinion the genes in the nuclei of cells still double themselves in this way. The most familiar analogy to the process is crystallization. A crystal grows if placed in a supersaturated solution, but the precise arrangement of the molecules out of several possible arrangements depends on the arrangement found in the original crystal with which the solution is "seeded." The metaphor of seeding, used by chemists, points to an analogy with reproduction.[116]

N. K. Koltzoff, the Russian cytogeneticist, also compared chromosomal duplication with that of crystallization.[117] For him the chromosome itself was a giant molecule having lateral chains, which were the genes. Duplication was a process of crystallization utilizing the building blocks of amino-acids and other chromosomal substances surrounding the chromosomes. Indeed, in his hypothesis the same process served not only to reproduce the chromosomes and their genic components but also additional gene copies that could then move to the cytoplasm to have their effects on development.

Sewall Wright also came to adopt the notion of gene as organism. In a review on the physiology of the gene written in 1941, Wright states: "The ultimate unit of life . . . is not the cell but the gene. . . . The data of genetic experiments directly imply the existence of numerous intracellular entities, each capable of synthesizing exact duplicates irrespective of the nature of the rest of the cell or of the organism or of the external environment, and producible only by such synthesis."[118]

The only qualification that Wright would have concerned mutation. Gene duplication was not absolutely perfect, and altered gene structures could arise through environmental action. But the environment did not specify the nature of the mutation, any more than it specified the kind of genic structure to be reproduced. The latter specification resided in the gene, even if it occasionally mutated, and this property is what Wright called *the autonomy of the genes*.

The point is repeated in an essay in 1948: "It is difficult to avoid the conclusion that the pattern of forces emanating from a gene somehow tends in the living cell to arrange simple molecules on its surface in such a way as to duplicate its molecular pattern."[119]

The idea of gene as organism was elaborated upon in his presidential address to the Society of American Naturalists in 1952.[120] In this thoughtful paper Wright developed an interesting concept of mind, applicable to different levels of organization in nature. For our present purposes, however, it is only relevant to note here that he recognized that entities at each of several levels of organization had the general properties justifying use of the common term organism, the properties, that is, of growth, development, reproduction, and adaptive change. The principles of integration of the component parts differed enormously in kind, of course, depending on whether the organism in question was a cell, a multicellular individual, or a society. However, the term "organism," Wright realized, often also connoted the notion of self-inclusiveness or self-dependence. Whether one considered genes, viruses, and DNA to be living would depend, therefore, upon the weight given to autonomy in the definition of organism. But autonomy was always a relative matter. For Wright, genes, viruses, and DNA were living if *autonomy of pattern* rather than metobolic independence were made the criterion.[121]

VI. Sequelae

By 1950 it was generally accepted among biologists that the gene had a physical reality and could somehow determine, even if not absolutely autonomously, both its own pattern during cell reproduction and specific metabolic events of cellular and organismal development. The principal purpose of this paper has been served by tracing the idea up to that time. Nevertheless, I shall try, in this section, to summarize somewhat sketchily some of the sequelae, in order to bring the situation up to date, before drawing conclusions from the history as I have understood it.

That a correlation existed between genes and enzymes was obviously clear to geneticists from the early years of the twentieth century. What was shown by the later experiments of the English group on flower pigments,[122] of Beadle and Ephrussi on transplantation in *Drosophila* larvae,[123] and of Beadle and Tatum on nutritional mutants in the mold *Neurospora,*[124] was the exquisite specificity of the gene: enzyme relationship. For each gene there was a specific, enzymatically catalyzed chemical reaction under its control. These findings of the late thirties and early forties suggested, but provided no proof for the suggestion, that each gene was responsible for the production of a distinct enzyme. The alternative possibility was still open: genes were transported to serve as enzymes in the cytoplasm. The improbability of this alternative was realized when the evidence became persuasive with the discovery of DNA as genetic transforming agent[125] and as the determiner of viral reproduction,[126] that DNA rather than protein was the material of which genes were composed.

Somewhat in advance of the acceptance of DNA as the genic material, however, new theories were already being proposed about the nature of gene duplication. In part, the new ideas were being created because the notion of attraction between identical molecules as the basis of autocatalytic reproduction of genes and viruses no longer seemed sound. In 1940 Linus Pauling and Max Delbrück published a short theoretical note in the journal *Science* asserting that the quantum-mechanical forces of resonance between identical molecules could not be large enough to cause attraction between like molecules under the conditions prevailing in living organisms. In that note Pauling and Delbrück offered the opinion

that the processes of synthesis and folding of highly complex molecules in the living cell involve, in addition to covalent-bond formation, only the intermolecular interactions of van der Waals attraction and repulsion, electrostatic interactions, hydrogen-bond formation, etc. which are now rather well understood. These interactions are such as to give stability to a system of two molecules with complementary structures in juxtaposition, rather than of two molecules with necessarily identical structure; we accordingly feel that complementariness should be given primary consideration in the discussion of specific attraction between molecules and the enzymatic synthesis of molecules.[127]

In part, too, new ideas were being generated as a result of new information about the structure of chromosomes. By 1940, the year Pauling and Delbrück were advancing the idea of complementariness as the primary cause of biological autocatalysis, the isolated chromosome had been shown to contain both protein and nucleic acid. In that year, H. Friederich-Freksa was also suggesting the interesting possibility of gene duplication through a structural complementarity between the nucleic acid and protein components of the chromosome.[128] The electrically positive nucleic acid portion was imagined to hold a structurally complementary and electrically negative protein on each side. The latter then served as a lattice on which the building-blocks of nucleic acid could be assembled according to a pattern determined by the existing structure. In this way, reproduction of the gene regarded as a nucleoprotein, could be accomplished, as well as synapsis between homologous chromosomes.

The notion of complementarity was also utilized by Sterling Emerson,[129] who saw in antigen-antibody and enzyme-substrate interactions a basis for gene reproduction. An antigen was supposed to possess a surface complementary to that of the specific antibody with which it forms a complex structure. Similarly, the substrate of an enzyme was believed to have a structure complementary to at least a portion of the catalyst. The gene might, therefore, possess a structure complementary to that of another molecule, and the latter might be instrumental in serving as a template for the construction of a new gene. The template might in fact be the enzyme that the gene specifies; if such were the case, the enzyme-template would be fully as autocatalytic as the gene. The latter possibility was entertained only because it provided a model at once for gene duplication and for gene specification of enzyme structure. Emerson's early experimental results[130] on the mutagenicity of antibodies directed against specific enzymes seemed to support the idea, but no evidence was subsequently reported of any *specific* mutagenicity with specific antibodies, and so the idea was dropped.

Models involving complementarity were, therefore, already in vogue prior to the report of Watson and Crick on the structure of DNA.[131] The significance of the Watson–Crick model, however, was that DNA alone was capable of serving as its own template for reproduction because of its bipartite structure. The two strands of the DNA double helix were complementary to each other because of base pairing restrictions between thymine and guanine and between guanine and cytosine. Each strand served as a template for its complement, and so the double helix was reproduced. The Watson–Crick model of DNA also, of course, had the great virtue of accounting for the then existing facts about DNA structure. In addition, it suggested a means for genetic determination of protein structure: the specific sequence of bases along one of the strands of DNA could serve as an encoded determiner of the *specific* sequence of amino-acids in a protein. The manner in which this suggestion emanating from the Watson–Crick model was elaborated upon and experimentally confirmed was truly one of the great scientific achievements of our time. A single-stranded messenger molecule of RNA, slightly different in its component parts from DNA, is now known to be constructed upon one strand of DNA serving as a template. The messenger is complementary to the template strand, which itself does not directly intervene in protein synthesis. The messenger makes its way to the cytoplasm where, in the complicated organelle called a ribosome, its sequence of bases orders the connecting together of the twenty different kinds of amino-acids into a polypeptide chain,[132] which then folds into a specific configuration determined by the amino-acid sequence. This specific configuration, in turn, determines the catalytic specificity of the polypeptide (or of the protein of which the polypeptide may become a part).

This theory of gene reproduction and gene action (as the control of enzyme production is called today) is the basis of modern molecular biology. It is also obviously a physicochemical embodiment of the distinction between the autocatalytic and heterocatalytic functions that Troland signaled. Today the language is changed, of course. The autocatalytic function of the gene is referred to as *replication*; the heterocatalytic function is combined in the *transcription* of DNA into an RNA messenger and in the *translation* of the latter into protein. Moreover, the operational separability of the autocatalytic and heterocatalytic functions is implicit in current theories of the *regulation* of gene action. In such models as those of Jacob and Monod,[133] for example, which explain the regulated synthesis of enzymes in bacteria, the gene may be replicated independently of its heterocatalytic expression. Genes may fail to be transcribed into messengers, or the messengers may fail to be translated, and yet the genes remain intact and capable of replication.

In modern parlance, what makes the gene a determinant is the unidirectional transfer of chemical information. This concept is what Crick only half-jokingly refers to as the "central dogma" of molecular biology:[134] DNA determines its own structure and that of RNA; RNA determines that of protein. Protein cannot *specify* the structures of genes. The arrow moves one way. In this sense, DNA is an organism, for it is the dictator of its own structural pattern.

In recent years this "central dogma" has been mildly shaken by only one critical argument and one empirical finding. The argument is that of Barry Commoner,[135] who objected to the idea of DNA as being a self-dependent determinant of its structure. He pointed out that protein enzymes are known to be necessary for both DNA replication and RNA transcription, as well as for protein synthesis. Perhaps, in fact, some of the specificity of DNA synthesis might be attributable to the enzymes (DNA polymerases) that catalyze the process. The rebuttal to such arguments usually consists in the demonstration that the DNA template is the determiner of the structural arrangement of the DNA product in syntheses conducted *in vivo,* however necessary DNA polymerases may be to make the syntheses proceed swiftly. Alternative forms of a DNA polymerase, which can influence the fidelity with which the DNA template is copied, are themselves determined by alternative forms of DNA.[136]

The finding that caused a slight stir in recent years was that of reverse transcriptase, an enzyme that catalyzes the synthesis of DNA using RNA rather than DNA as a template.[137] This enzyme is contained in certain animal-infecting viruses that contain RNA rather than DNA. With viral RNA serving as template and reverse transcriptase serving as catalyst, a DNA product complementary to the template can be produced *in vitro* from DNA building-blocks. This result was originally surprising, because it seemed to invalidate the "central dogma" of unidirectional flow of information from DNA. The result is no longer taken as a serious threat to the "dogma," however, as molecular biologists have adapted to it by altering their theoretic formulation: now the arrow can be shown in both directions between DNA and RNA, but it remains unidirectional between RNA and protein.[138] Thus, the argument goes that once information in the form of a molecular pattern is transmitted from nucleic acid (be it DNA or RNA) to protein, it cannot get out again. The molecular structure of nucleic acid remains determined by nucleic acid. In reality, the "central dogma" of molecular biology is a restatement, albeit in molecular language, of the denial of inheritance of acquired characters. The "central dogma" is a claim that the specificity with which a given (molecular) pattern is reproduced is owing to the preexistence of that pattern and not to the environment, which includes constituents (such as protein) resulting from the activity of that pattern.

VII. Conclusions

Just as nineteenth-century biology saw the replacement of Aristotle's final cause by the operation of natural selection, twentieth-century biology came to be marked by the materialization of his formal cause of generation. I have tried to show that this new view was due to an important distinction made in the early part of the century: a material substance was supposed to exist that possessed two distinct properties, reproducibility of form as well as activity in effecting some change in its environment. The two properties were not only conceptually but also operationally distinct; that is to say, the one property could be manifested without expression of the other. The distinction was hardly a trivial one, for many biologists at the turn of the century, and this group included Weismann, had difficulty conceiving of a material substance that was not altered and thus not consumed as a consequence of its activity. The realization that catalysts, including enzymes, are not consumed in the processes they catalyze,[139] must have been the basis for the initial speculation that the genetic material is catalytic. The second step was to create some physicochemically tenable model by which the catalyst was reproducible and its reproduction separate from its intervention in other chemical processes. This step was largely the work of Leonard Troland. Subsequent steps essentially involved a refinement of the physicochemical model, particularly in the further distinction between gene and enzyme. Nevertheless, the original distinction between the two properties of the genetic material remained.

The value of the distinction in the further progress of biology can hardly be gainsaid. That genes can be reproduced without intervening in development is now a guiding concept in the research of developmental biologists. What many investigators wish to discover today is how the developmental activity of the ever-present genes can be unleashed or repressed during individual ontogeny.[140] The distinction between the two properties of the hereditary material has also been useful in thinking about the meaning of organism. No longer is it commonly supposed that one can determine whether a thing is alive on the basis of its belonging to a particular level of organization. The dual properties that Troland called auto- and heterocatalytic have been observed at various levels of organization, and "life" is regarded as the manifestation of those properties. When multiple organisms at a given level manifest integrated heterocatalytic activities, so that a reproducible pattern is ascribable to the ensemble, an organism (or "individual") of a higher level of complexity is recognized. Organisms at no level of organization are entirely autonomous, however "free" or "self-dependent" they sometimes appear to be. Organisms are simply inconceivable without an environment, without a larger context with which to interact, and their "life" is not compatible with every conceivable environment. This is not to say that the distinction between "living" and "nonliving" has disappeared. We still find the concept of organism a useful and necessary one, even if an abstraction. It would be equally wrong to assume that biologists who view at least certain molecules as being alive are claiming to have "reduced" life to a molecular level. J. B. S. Haldane was an early exponent of a theory of the molecular origin of life, and yet he was cautious about any claim of reduction. By "mechanism" Haldane meant a "machine that depended upon its parts in order to function and that could not replace any lost or damaged parts.'' If organisms could be called machines at all, they had to be, to use Haldane's phrase, "self-regulating, self-repairing, and self-perpetuating machines,"[141] which certainly placed them in a class distinct from the kinds of man-made machines we are familiar with. Haldane summarized his view as follows:

Shakespeare's plays consist of words. . . . But the arrangement of the words is even more important than the words themselves. And in the same way life is a pattern of chemical processes. This pattern has special properties. It begets a similar pattern, as a flame does, but it regulates itself as a flame does not, except to a slight extent. . . . So when we have said that life is a pattern of chemical processes, we have said something true and important. . . . But to suppose that one can describe life fully on these lines is to attempt to reduce it to mechanism, which I believe to be impossible. On the other hand, to say that life does not consist of chemical processes is to my mind as futile and untrue as to say that poetry does not consist of words.[142]

As Sewall Wright has pointed out, organisms at different levels of organization exhibit their living properties in quite different ways. The means by which a society grows, reproduces and adapts are not identical to those by which a cell or a molecule of DNA may be said to do so. Our terms of description and our explanations differ to the extent that different component parts and processes are seen to be involved. Reduction, in the sense of providing a common, unified explanation of living phenomena, does not seem to be the goal of biologists who have accepted the possibility of "living" molecules.[143]

From a heuristic point of view, the new concept of organism has been of undoubted influence in scientific investigations of the origin of life. Following upon the theories of Troland, Muller, and particularly Haldane, the question is no longer being asked whether spontaneous generation of life from nonlife is a regular phenomenon in the present state of the earth. Rather, one asks how and under what conditions a "living" molecule might be engendered from a nonliving substrate.[144] Whether or not the first "living" molecule (if there ever was a "first") arose in the precise way imagined cannot be ascertained with certainty. If the imagined pathway proved to be effective in producing "living" molecules under man-made conditions, we would only know that the gap between the "nonliving" and the "living" can be bridged under certain conditions, conditions that may be rarely realizable in the absence of man's intervention.

The history of the concept I have been exploring in this article merits some reflections concerning the nature of scientific progress. In that history, metaphysical controversy, in particular, appears to have played a major role. There seems little doubt, for example, that the material and seemingly mechanical explanation of Weismann served as a challenge to Driesch, and that the vitalistic views of the latter incited scientists like Loeb,[145] Troland,

and Muller[146] to respond with new insights and observations. However much the mechanism vs. vitalism controversy appears interminable and to take on ever-new forms (as, for example, in reductionism vs. organicism or compositionism),[147] the controversy itself has stimulated fruitful work. Driesch's observations of the regulative capability of the embryo were valid and had to be explained even if the motive for the observations may have been to reject Weismann's model. In turn, the search for a causal relationship between genes and enzymes occurred as early as it did and led to useful theoretical distinctions primarily because of the hope on the part of contemporary biologists of rebutting Driesch's nonmaterial explanatory principles. The extent to which a metaphysical position orients a program of research may often be more hidden than it was in the case examined here. Yet the critical issues in a scientific field may never be joined without some strongly divergent ways of looking at the field itself. It may matter little that the opponent's position is poorly articulated or misunderstood; it is what the challenger understands by it that creates a will to find disconfirming evidence or a new theory. This hypothesis would account for the fact that despite the oft-reported deaths of vitalism and mechanism the battle between these hoary foes rages yet.[148] It would also explain why Lysenkoists in the Soviet Union rejected the theory of the gene. It is "idealistic" to hold the notion of a substance having a pattern that is reproduced in a manner largely independent of environmental variations, precisely because that notion appears to threaten the ordinary conception of interaction between material entities and components of their environment, to say nothing of the conception of "inheriting acquired characters."[149]

The history I have been unfolding offers us further instances of the usefulness of concepts embedded in erroneous contexts. Advance in scientific knowledge does not come about exclusively in the light of theories that prove infallible in every respect. It may have been unwise to equate the hereditary material with the enzyme of the organism as Troland and a number of biologists did in the early decades of the century. From our vantage point, this may seem to have been an unnecessary and erroneous step. We have the advantage today, however, of being able to distinguish between the protein enzymes that the organism is capable of making and the nucleic acid-genetic material upon which the making of these enzymes depends. Troland must not, obviously, be faulted for failing to know more about proteins and nucleic acids than was known at the time of World War I. One might also claim that equating genes with enzymes, instead of postulating enzymes to be products of gene action, was in the early years a proper exercise of Occam's razor. Until a more complicated hypothesis was required by the data, why not entertain the simpler one?

Moreover, the early equation between genes and enzymes appears to have been motivated, as I have suggested earlier, by the search for a physical model for the gene's properties. Very small amounts of catalyst are needed to effect catalysis; the catalyst is not immediately consumed by its action; catalysts are known to exist in cells. What better physical analogy for the gene, at a time when a physical analogy was desperately needed? Analogies may prove, as they usually do, faulty upon further analysis, but a least they get you moving in a new and possibly fruitful direction. The genius of Troland's theory lay primarily in the distinction he made between the autocatalytic or reproductive function of the germ plasm and the heterocatalytic capacity to facilitate selectively some chemical reaction other than self-synthesis. He assumed that particles of collodial dimensions and of the appropriate composition would have both of these properties. This assumption may easily be regarded as having been more important in the long run than a correct guess about the chemical nature of the particles themselves.

The significance of Troland's youthful contribution to genetic theory may be impossible to assess with finality. The valuable core of his theoretical insights probably would have been conceived by others if he had never existed or committed his thoughts to paper. Certainly, the core of Mendel's theory was re-created thirty-five years later in ignorance of that scientist's original work. Yet we do not appreciate Mendel the less for that. The fact is that Troland's theoretical papers in *The Monist* and *The American Naturalist* were known to biologists and they did have a remarkable influence, particularly upon H. J. Muller, who, if we are to judge from his notes for an unpublished treatise on the "Principles of Heredity," was undoubtedly moving in a similar direction. The confidence that Troland exhibited in physicochemical matters may have increased the credence of his theory in Muller's eyes, at least at the outset. Muller became more critical of Troland's naive views of catalysis, however, as time went by.

What emerges from this historical enquiry, in any case, is that an idea is not like a preexisting germ, encapsulated from very early times, remaining essentially unaltered in its passage from generation to generation. Were this true, the historian of science need only locate it intact, however disguised it may be, in the various historical contexts in which it may be found. Rather, an idea is at once the product and catalyst of our evolving knowledge and, as such, cannot be either constant or constantly in flux. It seems to me as incorrect to say that Aristotle's form is today's double helix as to suppose that the double helix is a revolutionary concept without intellectual precedent. The form and the helix are related, and it is instructive to discover how they are.

NOTES

1. Aristotle, *Generation of Animals*, trans. A. L. Peck (Cambridge, 1963), Book I, chapter 18, 722a,b.
2. W. Harvey, *On Animal Generation,* trans. R. Willis, *The Works of William Harvey* (London, 1847), p. 338.
3. A. Weismann, *Essays upon Heredity and Kindred Biological Problems* (Oxford, 1891).

The account given here does not pretend to give a chronological development of Weismann's views, but rather bears directly upon how those views relate to the principal theme of this essay.

4. A. Weismann, *The Germ Plasm*, trans, W. N. Parker and H. Rönnefeldt (New York, 1898).

5. The emboîtement version of preformationism, which arose in the seventeenth century, was of course not readily consistent with notions of inheritance of acquired characters; pangenetic versions like those of Empedocles, Anaxagoras, Democritus, Hippocrates, and Darwin, on the other hand, were.

6. Hippocrates, *Airs, Waters, Places*, trans. J. Chadwick and W. N. Mann, *The Medical Works of Hippocrates* (Oxford, 1950), p. 103.

7. Aristotle, *Generation of Animals*, Book I, chapter 17, 721b.

8. C. Darwin, *The Variation of Animals and Plants under Domestication*, 2nd rev. ed. (New York, 1876). chapter 27.

9. A Weismann, *Essays upon Heredity*.

10. A. Weismann, *Continuity of the Germ Plasm*, 1885, *Essays upon Heredity*, p. 170.

11. Ibid., p. 181.

12. Ibid., particularly pp. 187–88.

13. Ibid., p. 170.

14. Ibid., pp. 189–90.

15. A. Weismann, *On the Number of Polar Bodies and Their Significance in Heredity*, 1887, *Essays upon Heredity*.

16. A. Weismann, *Amphimixis or the Essential Meaning of Conjugation and Sexual Reproduction*, 1891; *Essays upon Heredity*.

17. A. Weismann, *The Germ Plasm*, chapter 12, p. 395.

18. Ibid., p. 395.

19. A. Weismann, *Continuity of the Germ Plasm*, p. 191.

20. H. De Vries, *Intracelluläre Pangenesis* (Jena, 1889); *Intracellular Pangenesis*, trans. C. S. Gager (Chicago, 1910).

21. De Vries's units were called *intracellular pangenes* to distinguish them from Darwin's pangenes that were capable of an intercellular existence and transport. De Vries did not require the postulate of intercellularity, since he accepted Weismann's refutation of inheritance of acquired characters. See Lindley Darden, *Reasoning and Scientific Change: The Field of Genetics at Its Beginnings*, Ph.D. Thesis, University of Chicago, 1974.

22. W. Roux, *Beiträge zur Entwicklungsmechanik des Embryo*, Virchow's Archiv. 114, (1888): 113–53, 246–91.

23. H. Driesch, *Entwicklungsmechanische Studien*. I–II. Zeits. Wiss. Zool. 53 (1891): 160–84; III–VI, ibid. 55 (1892): 1–62. Today Driesch's experiments may be properly criticized for failing to provide a critical test of the Weismannian hypothesis. To invalidate the hypothesis one must show that cells that have become somatically differentiated are still capable of giving rise to a normal organism. It is by no means obvious that the cells of the 4-cell stage, which Driesch used, are so differentiated; utilization of the chromosomes may not yet have occurred by that stage. It took the more recent work of J. B. Gurdon (*Nuclear transplantation in amphibia and the importance of stable nuclear changes in promoting cellular differentiation*, Quart, Rev. Biol. 38 [1963]: 54–78) to show that the Weismannian hypothesis is invalid.

24. H. Driesch, *The Science and Philosophy of the Organism* (London, 1908). Earlier publications were : *Analytische theorie der organischen Entwicklung* (Leipzig, 1894); *Die Localisation morphogenetischer Vorgange; ein Beiweis Vitalistischen Geschehens* (Leipzig, 1899); *Die organischen Regulationen* (Leipzig, 1901).

25. H. Driesch, *Science and Philosophy of the Organism*, p. 240.

26. Ibid., p. 142.

27. Ibid., p. 144.

28. T. Schwann, *Microscopische Untersuchungen über die Uebereinstimmung in der Strucktur und dem Wachstum der Tiere und Pflanzen*, trans. H. Smith, *Schwann and Schleiden Researches* (London 1847), p. 192.

29. Ibid., quoted by F. Jacob, *The Logic of Life* (New York, 1973), p. 119.

30. M. J. Schleiden, *Beiträge zur Phytogenese*, trans. H. Smith, *Schwann and Schleiden Researches* (London, 1847), p. 231.

31. C. Brücke, *Die Elementaroganismen*, Sitzungsbericht, Akad. der Wissenschaften 44 (Wien, 1861): 381–406.

32. A. Espinas, *Des Sociétés Animales, Etude de Psychologie Comparée* (Paris, 1877), p. 10.

33. H. Spencer, *Progress: Its Law and Cause* (New York, 1881), p. 269; *The Data of Ethics* (New York, 1884), chap. 8.

34. G. L. L. de Buffon, *Histoire naturelle*, 3rd ed., trans. W. Smellie (London, 1791), chapter 2.

35. E. B. Wilson, *The Cell in Development and Inheritance*, revised edition (New York, 1900), p. 291.

36. See Robert Kohler, *The background to Eduard Buchner's discovery of cell-free fermentation*, J. Hist. Biol. 4 (1971): 35–61; *The reception of Eduard Buchner's discovery of cell-free fermentation*, ibid. (1972): 327–53.

37. See J. S. Fruton, *Molecules and Life* (New York, 1972), particularly pp. 1–179.

38. An excellent account of the discovery and rediscovery of Mendelian theory is given in Robert C. Olby's *Origins of Mendelism* (New York, 1966).

39. An early report of Loeb's studies on heliotropism is contained in *Der Heliotropismus der Tiere und seine Uebereinstimmung mit dem Heliotropismus der Pflanzen* (Würzburg, 1889). Further references are contained in his lecture *The Significance of Tropisms for Psychology* collected in *The Mechanistic Conception of Life* (1912, reprinted by Harvard University Press, Cambridge, Mass., 1964).

40. Loeb originally controlled activation of already fertilized sea-urchin eggs through the ionic concentration of the medium (*Investigations in physiological morphology. III. Experiments in cleavage*, J. Morph. 7 [1892] 253–62), but later was able to produce normal pluteus larvae from unfertilized eggs (*On the nature of the process of fertilization*, Biological Lectures [1899]: 273–82).

41. J. Loeb, *On some facts and principles of physiological morphology*, Biological Lectures (1893): 37–62.

42. This argument was given in a footnote added to his Woods Hole Lecture of 1893 when it was reprinted in *The Mechanistic Conception of Life* (1912).

43. J. Loeb, *The recent development of biology*, Science 20 (1904): 777–86.

44. Ibid., p. 778.

45. J. Loeb, W. O. R. King, A. R. Moore, *Uber Dominanzerscheinungen bei den hybriden pluteen des Seeigels*, Roux' Archiv. f. Entw.-Mech. 29 (1907): 354–62.

46. A. R. Moore, *A biochemical conception of dominance*, U. Calif. Publications in Physiology 4 (1910): 9–15, *On Mendelian dominance*, Roux Archiv. f. Entw.-Mech. 34 (1912): 168–75. Moore received his Ph.D. from the University of California in 1911 and subsequently held professorial positions successively at California, Bryn Mawr, and Rutgers.

47. W. Bateson, *Mendel's Principles of Heredity* (Cambridge, 1909).

48. A. E. Garrod, *The incidence of alkaptonuria: a study in chemical individuality*, Lancet, 1902(2): 1616–20; *Inborn errors of metabolism*, ibid., 1908(2): 1–7, 73–79, 142–48, 214–20.

49. Bateson was using here an early form of the term *enzyme* or *intracellular catalyst*.

50. W. Bateson, *Mendel's Principles*, pp. 232–33.

51. Ibid., p. 268.

52. See note 46.

53. Moore rarely used the term "gene" or "allelomorph" in these papers, probably because he did not wish to preclude the possibility that the inherited factor is the enzyme.

54. Loeb devoted a chapter to enzymatic catalysis in *The Dynamics of Living Matter* (New York, 1906). In this chapter he emphasized, among other things, that biological catalysts may remain unaltered at the end of reactions in which they participate.

55. A. Lang, *Uber die Bastarde von Helix hortensis Mueller und Helix nemoralis L.* (Mit Beitraegen von Bosshard, Hesse und Kleiner). Festschrift d. Universitaet Jena, 1908.

56. A. R. Moore, *A biochemical conception of dominance*, pp. 14–15.

57. This is known as van't Hoff's rule. A discussion of this "rule" is to be found in Jan Bĕlhrádek's *Temperature and Living Matter* (Berlin, 1935).

58. J. Loeb and W. F. Ewald, *Die Frequenz der Herztätigkeit als eindentige Funktion der Temperatur*, Biochem. Ztschr. 58 (1913): 177–85.

59. J. Loeb and M. M. Chamberlain, *An attempt at a physico-chemical explanation of certain groups of fluctuating variation*, J. Exp. Zool. 19 (1915): 559–68, especially p. 560.

60. Ibid.

61. For a thorough account of Bateson's reluctance to accept a material description of the gene, see William Coleman's *Bateson and Chromosomes: Conservative Thought in Science*, Centaurus 15 (1970): 228–314.

62. E. M. East, *The Mendelian notation as description of physiological facts*, Amer. Nat. 46 (1912): 633–95. It is in this paper that East says that "Mendelism is . . . just such a conceptual notation as is used in algebra or in chemistry," and that "a Mendelian factor, not being a biological reality but a descriptive term, must be fixed and unchangeable."

63. It is an interesting sidelight on the role of prior intellectual commitment in scientific research to note that, where Loeb and Ewald in 1913 used the *similarity* of heartbeat in different *Fundulus* embryos as the basis for concluding hereditary control of enzymes, Loeb and Chamberlain two years later used the *variations* in segmentation rate between *Arbacia* eggs to conclude essentially the same thing.

64. H. Onslow, *A contribution to our knowledge of the chemistry of coat-colour in animals and dominant and recessive whiteness*, Proc. Roy. Soc. B. 89 (1915): 36–58.

65. S. Wright, *An intensive study of the inheritance of color and of other coat characters in guinea-pigs, with especial reference to graded variations*, Studies of Inheritance in Guinea-Pigs and Rats (W. E. Castle and S. Wright),II, Carnegie Inst. Wash. Publication No. 241 (1916).

66. R. Goldschmidt, *Genetic factors and enzyme reaction*, Science N. S. 43 (1916): 98–100; *Experimental intersexuality and the sex-problem* 50 (1916): 705–18.

67. R. Goldschmidt, *A further contribution to the theory of sex*, J. Exp. Zool. 22 (1917): 593–611.

68. Ibid., p. 595.

69. Ibid., p. 598.

70. O. Riddle, *Our knowledge of melanin color formation and its bearing on the Mendelian description of heredity*, Biol. Bull. 16 (1909): 316–50.

71. Ibid., pp. 324–25.

72. Ibid., pp. 339–40.

73. Ibid., pp. 344–45.

74. T. H. Morgan, A. H. Sturtevant, H. J. Muller, and C. B. Bridges, *The Mechanism of Mendelian Heredity* (New York, 1915).

75. Troland is a curious case in the history of science. Troland was an outsider to genetics. At least, his principal scientific contributions were outside that field, and he offered little else to either genetic, developmental or evolutionary biology after 1917. Trained in biochemistry as an undergraduate at M.I.T., he studied psychology for his doctoral degree, which he received from Harvard in 1915. He was entirely outside the mainstream of biology when he began as a graduate student to write on heredity and evolution. From studies of the psychology and physiology of vision, which he taught at Harvard until 1929, he turned to invention of processes of color photography. Many patents were issued in his name, and his work became the foundation of the Technicolor Corporation, of which he was research director from 1925 until the end of his life in 1932. He was only forty-three years old when he died of a freak accident, falling from a precipice on Mount Wilson while having his photograph taken by his wife.

76. He was to co-author with Daniel F. Comstock a semi-popular book on *The Nature of Matter and Electricity* (New York, 1917). While that of the junior author, Troland's contribution represented a major part of the book.

77. Troland refers to W. Ostwald, *Über die zeitlichen Eigenschaften der Entwicklungsvorgange, Vorträge und Aufsätze über Entwicklungs-mechanik des Organismus* (ed. W. Roux), Heft 5 (Leipzig, 1908). In a subsequent issue of the same journal (Heft 12, 1911), the Dutch geneticist Avend Hagedoorn was writing of *Autocatalytic substances: the determinants for the inheritable characters*.

78. L. T. Troland, *The chemical origin and regulation of life*, The Monist 24 (1914): 92–133.

79. Troland was specifically referring to Bergson's *Creative Evolution*, published in 1911.

80. L. T. Troland, *The chemical origin* (n. 78), pp. 97–98.

81. Ibid., p. 98.

82. Ibid., p. 104.

83. Ibid., p. 105.
84. Ibid., p. 110.
85. Ibid., p. 112.
86. Ibid., p. 128.
87. L. T. Troland, *Biological enigmas and the theory of enzyme action*, Amer. Nat. 51 (1917): 321–50.
88. Ibid., p. 327.
89. Troland's principal sources were W. Ostwald's *A Handbook of Colloid Chemistry*, English translation of 1915; J. W. Mellor's *Chemical Statistics and Dynamics*, 1914; W. Bayliss's *The Nature of Enzyme Action*, 1914; W. H. and W. L. Braggs's *X-Rays and Crystal Structure*, 1915; and I. Langmuir's papers in the Journal of the American Chemical Society, beginning in 1916.
90. L. T. Troland, *Biological enigmas* (n. 87), p. 333.
91. Ibid., p. 333.
92. Ibid., p. 339.
93. Ibid., p. 341.
94. Ibid., p. 342.
95. C. M. Child, *Senescence and Rejuvenation* (Chicago, 1915), pp. 11–12.
96. Ibid., pp. 11–12.
97. Troland drew heavily upon Bateson (*Mendel's Principles of Heredity*, 1909; *Problems of Genetics*, 1913) and the Morgan School (*Mechanism of Mendelian Heredity*, 1915).
98. L. T. Troland, *Biological enigmas* (n. 87), p. 340.
99. W. Johannsen, *Elemente der exakten Erblichskeitlehre* (Jena, 1909), pp. 123–24.
100. See Frederick B. Churchill, *William Johannsen and the genotype concept*, J. Hist. Biol. 7 (1974): 1–30.
101. T. H. Morgan, *The theory of the gene*, Amer. Nat. 51 (1917): 513–44; p. 514.
102. Ibid., p. 535. Morgan does not name any of the individuals who were rashly failing to keep the two sets of questions apart, but he may have had Goldschmidt in mind.
103. Parts of the first two chapters intended for this book, to have been co-authored with Edgar Altenburg, were printed in *Studies in Genetics, The Selected Papers of H. J. Muller* (Bloomington, 1962).
104. H. J. Muller, *Variation due to change in the individual gene*, Amer. Nat. 56 (1922): 32–50; reprinted in *Studies in Genetics*, pp. 176–77.
105. Ibid., p. 184.
106. Ibid., p. 186.
107. H. J. Muller, The gene as the basis of life, Proc. Int. Congr. Plant. Sci. 1 (1929): 897–921; reprinted in *Studies in Genetics*, p. 196.
108. Ibid., p. 199.
109. H. J. Muller, *The gene*, Proc. Roy. Soc. B 134 (1947): 1–37.
110. The important work of O. T. Avery, C. M. MacLeod, and M. McCarty identifying the transforming substance in pneumococci to be deoxyribonucleic acid (*Studies on the chemical nature of the substance inducing transformation of pneumococcal types. Induction of transformation by a desoxyribonucleic acid fraction isolated from pneumococcus Type III*, J. Exp. Med. 79 [1944] 137–58) had been published and was referred to in Muller's lecture.
111. Authoritative works at that time were, for example: *Proteins, Amino-acids and Peptides*, by Edwin J. Cohn and John T. Edsall (New York, 1943), and *Nucleic Acid* (Cambridge, 1947). In the case of both proteins and nucleic acids, a covalently bonded polymeric structure was envisaged. While the possibility of variant arrangements based on variation in the proportions of the different building-blocks was recognized in the case of proteins, the notion of an homogeneous, invariant nucleic acid molecule was to be overthrown only after the critical analyses of Erwin Chargaff (*Chemical specificity of nucleic acids and mechanism of their enzymatic degradation*, Experientia 6 [1950] 201–09).
112. R. M. Herriott, Q. R. Bartz, and J. H. Northrup, *Transformation of swine peptogen into swine pepsin by chicken pepsin*, J. Gen. Physiol. 21 (1938): 572–82.
113. H. J. Muller, *The gene* (n. 109), p. 19.
114. Originally published in the Rationalist Annual for 1928, the essay was reprinted in *The Inequality of Man* (London, 1932), and in *Science and Human Life* (New York, 1933).
115. J. B. S. Haldane, *The origin of life*, in *The Inequality of Man*, p. 156.

116. Ibid., pp. 156–57.

117. N. K. Koltzoff, *Physikalisch-chemische Grundlage der Morphologie.* Biol. Ztrbl. 48 (1928): 345–69; *The structure of the chromosomes and their participation in cell-metabolism*, Biol. J. 7 (1938): 3–46.

118. S. Wright, *The physiology of the gene*, Physiol. Rev. 21 (1941): 487–527; p. 487.

119. S. Wright, *Genes as physiological agents*, Amer. Nat. 79 (1948): 289–303; p. 294.

120. S. Wright, *Gene and organism,* Amer. Nat. 87 (1953): 5–18.

121. This is also probably what J. B. S. Haldane meant when, in his *Origin of life* article cited above (p. 147, 1933 reprint), he wrote as follows: "In the present state of our ignorance we may regard the gene either as a tiny organism which can divide in the environment provided by the rest of the cell; or as a bit of machinery which the 'living' cell copies at each division. The truth is probably somewhere between these two hypotheses."

122. The work, in particular, by M. Wheldale (later Mrs. Onslow), R. Robinson, W. J. C. Lawrence, and R. Scott-Moncrieff was reviewed in R. Scott-Moncrieff, *A biochemical survey of some Mendelian factors for flower color*, J. Genetics 32 (1936): 117–70; and *The genetics and biochemistry of flower color variation*, Ergeb. Enzymforsch. 8 (1939): 277–306.

123. G. W. Beadle and B. Ephrussi, *Development of eye colors in Drosophila: Diffusible substances and their interrelations*, Genetics 22 (1937): 76–86.

124. G. W. Beadle and E. L. Tatum, *Genetic control of biochemical reactions in Neurospora*, Proc. Nat Acad. Sci. U.S. 27 (1941): 499–506. Their work and that of the school that developed in response to the initial discoveries of biochemical mutants in *Neurospora* were reviewed by G. W. Beadle, *Genetics and metabolism in Neurospora*, Physiol. Rev. 25 (1945): 643–63.

125. O. T. Avery, C. M. MacLeod, and M. McCarty, *Studies* (n. 110). There has been some recent questioning of the extent to which geneticists were aware of this important work. That leading geneticists were definitely appreciative of the broad significance of the studies on pneumococcal transformation is evidenced not only by Muller's reference to this work (see above) but also by the early reference made to it, even in advance of its definitive publication, by Th. Dobzhansky in the second edition of his classic work on *Genetics and the Origin of the Species* (New York, 1941), pp. 47–50.

126. A. D. Hershey and M. Chase, *Independent functions of viral protein and nucleic acid in growth of bacteriophage*, J. Gen. Physiol. 36 (1952): 39–56.

127. L. Pauling and M. Delbrück, *The nature of the intermolecular forces operative in biological processes*, Science 92 (1940): 77–79. This note was obviously in reaction to earlier suggestions by P. Jordan (*Zum Frage einer spezifischen Anziehung zwischen Genmolekülen*, Phys. Zeits. 39 [1938]: 711–14; *Uber quantenmechanische Resonanz-anziehung und über das Problem der Immunitätsreaktionen*, Zeits. f. Phys. 113 [1939] 431–38; *Zum problem der spezifischen Immunität*, Fundam. Radiol. 15 [1939]: 43–46) that the quantum-mechanical resonance phenomenon could account for attraction between molecules of identical structure and to the autocatalytic reproduction of molecules. Pauling and Delbrück's counterproposal of complementarity refers to a "fit" between the three-dimensional configurations of a pair of molecules allowing them to approach each other sufficiently to form bonds of either a weak or stable nature. It is in this sense that the molecular biologist today regards the reactant in an enzymatically catalyzed reaction to be complementary to at least a part of the enzyme, as is an antigen to its antibody.

128. H. Friederich-Freksa, *Bei der Chromosomenkonjugation wirksame Kräfte und ihre Bedeutung für die identische Verdopplung von Nucleoproteinen*, Naturwiss. 28 (1940): 376–79.

129. S. Emerson, *Genetics as a tool for studying gene structure*, Ann. Miss. Bot. Garden 32 (1944): 179–83.

130. S. Emerson, *The induction of mutations by antibodies*, Proc. Nat. Acad. Sci. U.S. 30 (1945): 243–49.

131. J. D. Watson and F. H. C. Crick, *A structure for deoxyribonucleic acid,* Nature 171 (1953): 737–38; *Genetic implications of the structure of deoxyribonucleic acid*, Ibid., pp. 964–67.

132. A polypeptide chain is a molecule containing a specific, unique sequence of amino-acids covalently bonded to each other through so-called peptide bonds. We know today that many

proteins are composed of one or more such chains. When proteins consist of two or more chains, the latter may be identical or different. A given (structural) gene specifies the amino-acid sequence of a particular polypeptide.

133. F. Jacob and J. Monod, *Genetic regulatory mechanisms in the synthesis of proteins*, J. Mol. Biol. 3 (1961): 318–56.

134. F. H. C. Crick, *Central dogma of molecular biology*, Nature (Lond.) 227 (1970): 561–63, Unfortunately, the term "central dogma" is poorly chosen, since the assertion it makes is not without experimental support and would be rejected if empirically warranted.

135. B. Commoner, *DNA and the chemistry of inheritance*, Amer. Sci. 52 (1964): 365–88; *Failure of the Watson–Crick theory as a chemical explanation of inheritance*, Nature (Lond.) 220 (1968): 334–40.

136. For a critique of Commoner's argu...ent, see P. Fleischman, *The chemical basis of inheritance*, Nature (Lond.) 225 (1970): 30–32; and A. D. Hershey, *Genes and hereditary characteristics*, Nature (Lond.) 226 (1970): 697–700.

137. D. Baltimore, *Viral RNA-dependent DNA polymerase*, Nature (Lond.) 226 (1970): 1209–11; H. M. Temin and S. Mizutani, *RNA-dependent DNA polymerase in virions of Rous sarcoma virus*, Nature (Lond.) 226 (1970): 1211–13.

138. For a discussion of the implications of reverse transcriptase on the "central dogma," see F. E. Hahn, *Reverse transcription and the central dogma*, Progress in Molecular and Subcellular Biology 3 (1973): 1–14.

139. At least not at a great rate. Today we realize that enzymes are not permanently unaffected by the catalysis they effect; while they are eventually consumed, their lifetimes are large considering the number of substrate molecules they "turn over."

140. See, for example, E. H. Davidson, *Gene Activity in Early Development* (New York, 1968), E. W. Hanley, ed., *Problems in Biology: RNA in Development* (Salt Lake City, 1970); and J. B. Gurdon, *The Control of Gene Expression in Animal Development* (Cambridge, 1974).

141. J. B. S. Haldane, *What Is Life?*, *Adventures of a Biologist* (New York, 1937), p. 52.

142. J. B. S. Haldane, *What Is Life?* (New York, 1947), p. 56.

143. See also D. L. Hull, *Reduction in genetics—biology or philosophy?* Phil. Sci. 39 (1972): 491–99.

144. Many books and symposia have been devoted in recent years to the "origin of life" problem. A few suggested readings are: A. I. Oparin, *The Origin of Life on the Earth,* 3rd rev. ed. (London, 1957); D. H. Kenyon and G. Steinman, *Biochemical Predestination* (New York, 1969); L. E. Orgel, *The Origins of Life* (New York, 1973).

145. The origins of Loeb's mechanistic position and the relation between his philosophical outlook and his scientific work are admirably discussed in Donald Fleming's Introduction to the 1964 reprint of Loeb's *The Mechanistic Conception of Life* by Harvard University Press.

146. Some indication of the interaction between Muller's scientific and philosophical views is available in E. O. Carlson, *The legacy of Hermann Joseph Muller: 1890–1967*, Canad. J. Gen. Cyt. 9 (1967): 436–48; T. M. Sonneborn, *H. J. Muller, crusader for human betterment*, Science 162 (1968): 772–76; G. E. Allen, *Science and society in the eugenic thought of H. J. Muller*, Bio Science 20 (1970): 346–53.

147. For an incisive discussion of the controversy see chapter 5 of D. L. Hull, *The Philosophy of Biological Science* (Englewood Cliffs, N.J., 1974).

148. See, for example, F. H. C. Crick: "... I believe the motivation of many of the people who have entered molecular biology from physics and chemistry has been their desire to *disprove* vitalism." *Of Molecules and Men* (Seattle, 1966), p. 24.

149. The metaphysical basis of Lysenkoist objections to gene theory is most apparent in Trofim Lysenko's *The Science of Biology Today* (New York, 1948). This is a translation of Lysenko's presidential address delivered at the famous session of the Lenin Academy of Agricultural Sciences of the U.S.S.R. in July 1948. It also appears in the complete proceedings of this session, *The Situation in Biological Science* (Moscow, 1949).

Experiment and Explanation in the Physiology of Bichat and Magendie

William Randall Albury

Part I: Experiment

INTRODUCTION. The scientific portraits of Xavier Bichat (1771–1802) and François Magendie (1783–1855) that have been preserved for us by the traditions of the historiography of physiology, have remained almost as sharply and simply drawn as when they first emerged from the hand of Claude Bernard. With his eulogy of Magendie in 1856, Bernard produced an evaluation of the scientific contributions of these two men, and of the relationship between their work, which he continued to expound throughout his career and which has been substantially followed by most historians of physiology ever since.[1] Bichat, we are told, was primarily a systematizer whose anatomical study of the tissues and occasional physiological experiments were largely vitiated by his adherence to a vitalistic theory of life. Magendie, on the other hand, is represented to us as a pure experimentalist who harbored a positivistic distrust of all theories and systems. Given these portraits of the two men, the relationship between their work is easily expressed: Magendie attacked the theoretical vitalism of Bichat and, having overthrown it, established in its place the experimental method. In other words, the vitalism of Bichat is understood as a conceptual obstacle to the progress of physiology—an obstacle that Magendie had to subject to a theoretical critique before he could found a truly experimental physiology.

The adequacy of this account becomes suspect, however, as soon as one considers the asymmetry of the relationship it proposes to establish, setting Magendie's methodology (experimentalism) against Bichat's explanatory sys-

William Randall Albury, School of History and Philosophy of Science, University of New South Wales.

tem (vitalism). Our curiosity is aroused as to the missing terms, about which little has been written: Bichat's methodology (for Bichat also performed experiments) and Magendie's explanatory system (for Magendie was also a vitalist). To what extent has the omission of these terms distorted our understanding of the relationship between the physiology of Bichat and Magendie? One distortion caused by an excessive concentration upon Magendie's criticisms of Bichat's theoretical position has been the failure to note that throughout the early part of his career Magendie frequently exhibited admiration for Bichat's experiments. In his doctoral thesis of 1808 Magendie quoted, in support of one of his own contentions, a lengthy passage from Bichat's *Traité d'anatomie descriptive* relating the latter's experiments on the production of sound by the larynx.[2] This same treatise was also cited several times by Magendie in the textbook of physiology which he published in 1816–17.[3] And despite his theoretical criticisms, Magendie still retained a high regard for his predecessor's "observing mind, his experimental genius," in the 1820s when he published annotated editions of Bichat's *Recherches physiologiques* and *Traité des membranes*.[4]

This observation raises the question, on which the first part of our study will focus, of the relationship between the methodologies of Bichat and Magendie. What were the similarities and differences between the experimental researches of these two men? To begin the investigation of this question we propose to examine an early research memoir of Magendie's, comparing the experiments reported in it with a number of experiments that had previously been carried out by Bichat. In this way we shall be able to determine whether the two men differed substantially at the level of experimental technique, and we shall also have a concrete point of reference for the subsequent methodological discussion. In the course of that discussion, which will complete the first part of our study, we shall examine the connection between Bichat's vitalistic theories and his overall method of physiological research in order to discover whether it was, in fact, his vitalism that posed the conceptual obstacle to the introduction of the experimental method in physiology. This inquiry will also enable us to characterize adequately the fundamental difference between the experiments of Bichat and those of Magendie, so that the theoretical foundations of that difference can be explored in the second part of this study when we turn our attention to the question of physiological explanation. Magendie's criticisms of Bichat's explanatory system, as well as his own suggestion for an alternative system of explanation, will be closely considered in part two; and we shall attempt to account for this difference in theoretical position in a way which will also illuminate the origins of the experimental method in physiology.

THE MEMOIR ON ABSORPTION. Our first task is to look carefully at the experimental techniques of Bichat and Magendie, and we shall begin this investigation by examining the most important memoir in the series of three that resulted from Magendie's first experimental researches in physiology. This series of memoirs was presented to the *Académie des sciences* of the *Institut de France* by Magendie and his collaborator, an otherwise obscure medical student named Robert Delille, between April and August of 1809.[5] The experiments reported in the first and third memoirs concerned the physiological effects of certain vegetable poisons, chiefly the strychnine forms *upas tieuté* and *upas antiar,* while the second memoir investigated the means by which these poisons were absorbed into the mammalian body.

It is the second memoir from this series, the one on absorption, which we shall examine here. Two factors recommend it for study, the first being that it described the most elaborate and impressive experiments of the series. Reviewing them more than half a century later, Claude Bernard told his students that these experiments were still as important as they had been when Magendie initially performed them.[6]

The second reason in favor of studying the memoir on absorption is that it was the only one of the series that Magendie chose to publish. All three memoirs were summarized in various publications in 1809, but Magendie himself printed the entire text of the second memoir in his own journal in 1821, with a note saying, "Although this work is eleven years old, I see with satisfaction that there is nothing in it that I have to change."[7] Thus the memoir on absorption not only affords us a sample of Magendie's earliest experimental researches, but it can also be taken as representative of his methodological and theoretical position at a later date.

The object of this memoir was to determine whether all substances—foreign materials as well as ingested food—were absorbed into the body by means of the lymphatic system alone, or whether some substances were absorbed directly by the venous system. The accepted opinion at the time held that absorption was carried out entirely by the lymphatics; indeed Bichat, as Claude Bernard observed, "took the expressions 'lymphatic system' and 'absorbent system' as synonymous."[8] Magendie, on the other hand, was led to assert that the venous system was sometimes the agent of absorption. At this level, then, we have an apparently simple contrast between Bichat and Magendie, and we shall return to the question of their differing conclusions about absorption somewhat later.

Our immediate concern, however, is to examine the series of experiments that led Magendie to his conclusion about absorption and to compare them with a series of experiments from the works of Bichat. But which of Bichat's experiments shall we choose for this purpose? He performed none on venous absorption; Magendie's experiments were "the first researches on this subject."[9] Rather than taking subject-matter as our guide, then, we shall select experiments from the works of Bichat that exhibit a certain degree of "structural similarity" with those described in Magendie's memoir.[10] In this way we shall be able to determine whether Magendie's researches on absorption represented an innovation in experimental technique or whether they merely applied existent procedural forms to a new area of inquiry.

EXPERIMENT I. Magendie became interested in the subject of absorption when he observed—as related in his first memoir[11]—that injected vegetable poisons were very rapidly absorbed into the circulatory system. The received explanation of this process was that foreign substances were conveyed through the lymphatic vessels to the thoracic duct, where they entered the bloodstream through the connections of this duct with the left subclavian vein. But since the lymphatic system, as Magendie noted, was chiefly characterized by the weakness and slowness of its action, the speed with which the poisons were absorbed into the blood cast doubt upon the adequacy of the accepted doctrine. Nevertheless, Magendie claimed that his experiments on the absorption of foreign substances were not undertaken with the intention of discovering new facts, but merely "to add a degree of certainty to an admitted explanation."[12] Thus his first experiment was to some extent a repetition of one that had recently been performed by the surgeon Guillaume Dupuytren (1777–1835) to study the absorption of chyle from ingested food.

Dupuytren had tied the thoracic duct in horses and had discovered that in those animals that lived more than five or six days after this operation some connection was always found between the lower part of the thoracic duct and the subclavian vein, allowing the chyle from the intestines to bypass the ligature. In those animals that died during the first week no such alternative connection could be found, hence their death by starvation. It had previously been known that some animals survived the ligature of the thoracic duct while others did not, and Dupuytren's findings explained this seeming anomaly; thus they supported the accepted doctrine of absorption by showing that an apparent exception to the rule of lymphatic absorption was in fact explicable by means of that rule.[13]

Magendie, attempting a similar experiment on dogs, had in mind the somewhat different question: "Would the ligature of the thoracic duct prevent the passage of the poison [*upas tieuté*] into the sanguinary system?"[14] Each time this poison was injected into the muscles or body cavities of an animal whose thoracic duct had been tied, the unmistakable toxic effects of the poison—violent tetanic convulsions and consequent death by asphyxiation—appeared as rapidly and as forcefully as they had when the thoracic duct was not ligatured. This result, however, as Magendie quickly pointed out, in no way proved that the poison was not carried by the lymphatic system, since the lymphatics could have had other points of communication with the circulatory system in addition to the thoracic duct. But unlike Dupuytren, Magendie did not attempt to demonstrate the existence of these connections in each of his animals by anatomical examination.[15]

Now although Magendie's first experiment on the absorption of foreign substances is related to Dupuytren's experiment on the absorption of nutriments, it nevertheless bears comparison with one of Bichat's most famous experiments as well: the demonstration in his *Recherches physiologiques* that the change in the color of the blood from black to red takes place during its transit through the lungs.[16] First of all it should be noted that Bichat, like Magendie, did not propose to discover new phenomena but only to give the added weight of experimental demonstration to an accepted view: "It is generally known that the blood is colored in passing through the lungs, that from the black that it was it becomes red; but until now this interesting matter has not been the object of any precise and rigorous experiment."[17]

By using two stop-cocks, the first fitted to the trachea of a dog and the second to one of the animal's major arteries, Bichat could simultaneously control the animal's respiration and produce a regulated flow of arterial blood in which any change of color could be observed. Whenever the tracheal stop-cock was shut the arterial blood was seen to change from red to black, the time required for this change being directly proportional to the amount of air contained in the lungs when the stop-cock was closed.[18] Hence the procedure of Bichat's experiment was to prevent the reddening of the blood (the effect of the entry of oxygen into the blood) by obstructing the trachea (the conduit through which the oxygen reaches the lungs)—thus showing, if successful, that oxygen enters the blood through the lungs.[19]

From this discussion of Bichat's experiment it can easily be seen that the procedure involved was essentially the same as that of Magendie's experiment. Magendie proposed to prevent the tetanic convulsions (the effect of *upas* entering the blood) by obstructing the thoracic duct (the conduit through which the *upas* was thought to reach the subclavian vein)—thus showing, if successful, that *upas* enters the blood through the subclavian vein. The experiments of Bichat and Magendie, then, are formally equivalent, as Table 1 shows.

TABLE 1

Experiment 1
Procedure: To prevent the entry of a substance into the circulatory system by obstructing the conduit conveying the substance to its supposed site of entry.

	Bichat	Magendie
substance	oxygen	*upas*
source	respiration	injection
conduit	trachea	thoracic duct
site of entry	lungs	subclavian vein
effect of entry	reddening of blood	tetanic convulsions, death
result	effect prevented	effected not prevented

Since Bichat's procedure did, in fact, prevent the effect in question from occurring—the reddening of the blood did cease when the trachea was obstructed—he next studied the reverse process: the reddening of arterial blood that had been blackened by asphyxiation. In this experiment he found that the blood changed almost immediately from black to red, without passing through gradations of color, when the tracheal stop-cock was opened. Magendie would undoubtedly have attempted an equivalent experiment had the ligature of the thoracic duct been found to prevent the symptoms of *upas* poisoning; but since the symptoms did appear, he had no reason to proceed in this manner.

Nevertheless, there is a final important point of comparison to be noted between Bichat's study of the coloring of blood by oxygen and Magendie's study of absorption; from his experiment on the reddening of previously blackened arterial blood, Bichat concluded as follows: "The rapidity with which the blood becomes red again when the stop-cock is opened scarcely permits any doubt that the principle which serves for this coloring passes directly from the lungs into the blood through the membranous walls of the [pulmonary] chambers, and that any longer route, such as that of the absorbent [i.e., lymphatic] system, for example, cannot be traversed by it."[20] Here we observe that Bichat based his conclusion on exactly the same point that Magendie said first struck him in his initial experiments on *upas*: the difficulty of the lymphatic system serving as the route for a very rapid absorption. Indeed, this difficulty may have been suggested to Magendie by Bichat's remark; for when Magendie discovered that the immediate cause of death in cases of *upas* poisoning is asphyxiation,[21] he would probably have consulted the relevant sections of Bichat's *Recherches physiologiques*, which were still recognized at the time as the foremost study of the subject.[22]

EXPERIMENT 2. Since Magendie's first experiment, involving the ligature of the thoracic duct, was inconclusive, he turned to another one that he hoped would produce "less equivocal results."[23] In this experiment he isolated a portion of a dog's small intestine between two ligatures by cutting all the lymphatic vessels and four each of the five mesenteric arteries and five mesenteric veins connected to it. Then the intestine itself was cut just beyond each of the ligatures, so that the only communication between the isolated loop and the rest of the body was through the single remaining mesenteric artery and vein; finally, even the "cellular coating" of these two vessels was removed, "for fear that lymphatics might be concealed within it."[24] When *upas* was injected into this isolated loop of intestine, however, the characteristic symptoms appeared with the same speed and force as they did when the poison was injected into a normal intestine.

This experiment, repeated several times, proved, wrote Magendie, "as much as one can prove in physiology, that the lacteal vessels [which are a part of the lymphatic system] are not the exclusive organs of intestinal absorption."[25] Nevertheless, he continued, this nonlymphatic mode of absorption might be peculiar to the intestines, and further researches would be required to determine whether it occurred in other parts of the body.

Before considering these further researches, let us turn once again to the works of Bichat to discover whether they contain an experiment comparable to the one just described. Such an experiment can indeed be found in Bichat's *Traité des membranes,*[26] and it bears the same relationship to the experiment on the reddening of blood in the lungs as Magendie's experiment on the intestinal loop bears to the one on the thoracic duct. The reason why Bichat's experiment on the intestinal loop was not included in the *Recherches physiologiques* is that the experiments in that book were devoted entirely to the functions of the brain, heart, and lungs.[27] In the *Traité des membranes,* however, the experiment on the intestine made up part of the study of the functions of the mucous membranes, since it is this type of membrane that forms the intestinal lining.

The question in which Bichat was interested was "whether the mucous membranes have any influence upon the redness of the blood"; that is, whether they "carry out functions accessory to those of the lungs."[28] In order to investigate this matter Bichat placed a ligature on the small intestine of a dog and then, through an opening made in another part of the intestine, inflated it with air from the opening to the ligature; after this, a second ligature was quickly placed between the first one and the opening so that an uncut portion of intestine was kept inflated with air by the two ligatures. An hour later Bichat examined the blood in the mesenteric veins leading from the inflated portion of the intestine and the blood in the other mesenteric veins to see whether there was any difference in color. Finding none, he repeated the experiment using pure oxygen instead of air and finally arranged matters so that the oxygen could be kept in motion through the intestinal loop, but in no case could he detect any reddening of the venous blood flowing from the loop.[29]

It is apparent that the procedure involved in this experiment by Bichat is the same as that found in Magendie's second experiment on absorption. Once again there is a formal equivalence that can be simply illustrated by means of Table 2.

Just as Magendie was unwilling to generalize from the results of his experiment on intestinal absorption to the mode of absorption occurring in other parts of the body, so too Bichat pointed out that one could not conclude from his experiment on the intestines that oxygen does not pass into the blood through other mucous membranes, because "although analogous, their organization could be different."[30] In the case of the other mucous membranes,

TABLE 2

Experiment 2

Procedure: To produce an effect showing that a substance within an isolated part of the body has entered the circulatory system.

	Bichat	Magendie
substance	oxygen	*upas*
source	injection	injection
isolated part	intestine	intestine
site of entry	mesenteric vein	mesenteric vein
effect of entry	reddening of blood	tetanic convulsions, death
result	effect not produced	effect produced

however, an experiment of the sort performed on the intestine could not be carried out, since the veins leading from them could not be examined. Hence the question had to be left unresolved, although Bichat related certain observations which suggested that none of these other membranes was permeated by oxygen either.[31]

Magendie, however, was not restricted to a consideration of mucous membranes, and he was thus free, as Bichat was not, to attempt on other parts of the body the same experimental procedure as that performed on the intestine. Selecting, for this attempt, the hind leg of a dog, he carefully separated it from the body (having previously sedated the animal with opium) so that only the crural artery and vein were left intact (see Fig. 1). After removing, once again, the "cellular coating" of these vessels, he injected *upas* into the foot and found that the usual effects of the poison appeared in exactly the same manner as when the leg was entirely connected to the body. Finally, to counter the possible objection that the arterial and venous walls themselves might contain tiny lymphatic vessels, Magendie cut each of these blood vessels, reconnecting them by means of hollow feather-shafts so that only the two columns of flowing blood united the leg with the body of the dog. But even under these circumstances the results of the injection were the same as before.[32]

Now it is clear that, apart from the refinement of the feather-shafts, this experiment on the dog's leg was simply the application to a different anatomical area of the previous experiment on the intestinal loop. Thus, as the following table shows, it was in all essential respects isomorphous with that previous experiment and with Bichat's experiment on the intestine as well.

With the success of the experiment on the dog's leg, Magendie had demonstrated the existence of venous absorption in other parts of the body as well as in the intestines. "This new mode of absorption" he concluded, "much more direct than the lymphatic absorption, provides the means for easily conceiving the rapidity with which various materials, harmful or otherwise, are absorbed, as well as the promptitude of the production of their effects in the [animal]

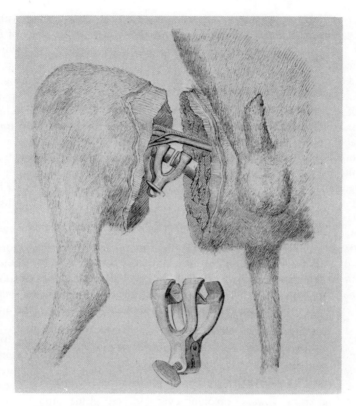

Fig. 1. Claude Bernard's illustration of the preparation of a dog's leg for Magendie's experiment on absorption (with metal clamp added); from C. Bernard, *Physiologie opératoire,* p. 337. (The photograph was supplied by Ms. Doris Thibodeau, Librarian of The Johns Hopkins Institute of the History of Medicine, and is reproduced here by permission of the Director of the Institute.)

TABLE 3

Experiment 2

Procedure: To produce an effect showing that a substance within an isolated part of the body has entered the circulatory system.

	Bichat	Magendie (A)	Magendie (B)
substance	oxygen	*upas*	*upas*
source	injection	injection	injection
isolated part	intestine	intestine	leg
site of entry	mesenteric vein	mesenteric vein	crural vein
effect of entry	reddening of blood	tetanic convulsions, death	tetanic convulsions, death
result	effect not produced	effect produced	effect produced

economy.''[33] He noted that his experiments did not rule out the possibility that tiny lymphatic capillaries might convey the *upas* from its place of entry into the body to nearby sanguinary capillaries and thus serve as intermediaries in the introduction of the poison into the venous system. Like Bichat, he had attained a limit beyond which his experiments could not reach. Nevertheless, he argued that experimental evidence already produced weighed heavily in favor of direct absorption by the veins.[34] Thus he felt justified in concluding ''that the lymphatic vessels are not always the route followed by foreign materials to reach the sanguinary system.''[35]

At this point it would appear that Magendie had adequately accounted for the rapid absorption of *upas*, the phenomenon which initially prompted his investigation. He could, then, have reasonably terminated his memoir here. Instead of doing this, however, he turned his attention to a related but distinct subject.

EXPERIMENT 3. Having shown that the blood of an animal suffering from the effects of *upas* must contain some amount of the poison, or, in other words ''that this blood is veritably poisoned,'' Magendie raised the question of ''whether this blood, introduced into the circulatory system of a healthy animal, would produce effects similar to those which it causes in the animal itself.''[36]

To investigate this matter Magendie first transfused arterial blood from a poisoned animal showing evident effects of the *upas* into the jugular vein of a normal animal. Although this operation ''lasted more than twenty minutes, so that the healthy animal received a very considerable quantity of poisoned blood,''[37] no signs of *upas* poisoning ever appeared in the animal receiving the blood. Such an unexpected result, Magendie offered, might suggest that the respiration of the first animal had somehow changed the nature of the *upas* so that while poisonous in the venous system it became harmless in the arterial system. But this suggestion was quickly overturned by two additional experiments in which venous blood was transfused. In the first, blood was taken from the left jugular vein of a dog three mintues after the animal had been stabbed in the left cheek with a sliver of wood soaked in *upas*.[38] In the second experiment the hind leg of a dog was isolated and injected, as in the earlier procedure, and blood was transfused from the crural vein into the jugular vein of a healthy animal ''for over ten minutes, more than enough time for the production of the effects of *upas*.''[39] Nevertheless, none of the animals receiving transfusions ever showed the characteristic signs of poisoning by *upas*. Hence Magendie was led to conclude that the blood of animals suffering from the effects of *upas* ''cannot produce fatal accidents in other animals.'' He ventured no explanation of this anomalous result, however, closing his memoir with the assertion that ''in the physiological sciences one should be frugal with conjectures and prodigal with facts.''[40]

Setting aside any concern with the outcome of Magendie's transfusion experiments and considering only their formal structure, we once again find equivalent experiments in Bichat's study of respiration and asphyxiation. In the second part of the *Recherches physiologiques,* during the course of his investigation of the phenomena of asphyxiation, Bichat showed that the primary effect of black blood passing without alteration through the lungs from the venous system into the arterial system was a loss of consciousness caused by the penetration of this blood into the capillaries of the brain.[41] To demonstrate this effect Bichat injected into the carotid artery of a dog some blood taken from its jugular vein, the consequence of which was that the dog developed the symptoms of asphyxiation.[42] Hence, he concluded, ''We are already authorized, I believe, to think that in asphyxia the circulation, which continues for some time after the chemical functions of the lungs have ceased, interrupts the function of the brain by conveying black blood to it through the arteries.''[43]

Here Bichat had made his point, and he could reasonably have passed on to other matter. Instead, however, he continued in a manner similar to that which we have seen at the end of Magendie's memoir: ''If in asphyxia the black blood suspends the cerebral action by its contact, then it is clear that opening an artery—for example the carotid—in an animal which is asphyxiated, taking the fluid from it, and injecting it gently into another animal in the direction of

TABLE 4

Experiment 3

Procedure: To demonstrate the effects of a substance in the circulatory system by transfusing that substance from the circulatory system of one animal into the circulatory system of another animal to produce those effects in the second animal.

	Bichat (A)	Magendie (A)	Magendie (B)
substance	black arterial blood	blood containing *upas*	blood containing *upas*
source in donor	asphyxiation	injection	injection
transfusion { from	carotid artery	arterial system	jugular vein
transfusion { into	carotid artery	jugular vein	venous system
effect on recipient	unconsciousness, death	tetanic convulsions, death	tetanic convulsions, death
result	effect produced	effect not produced	effect not produced
	Bichat (B)	Magendie (C)	
substance	black arterial blood	blood containing *upas*	
source in donor	asphyxiation	injection	
transfusion { from	carotid artery	crural vein	
transfusion { into	crural vein	jugular vein	
effect on recipient	paralysis, insensitivity of leg	tetanic convulsions, death	
result	effect produced	effect not produced	

the brain, ought to cause this latter animal to die equally asphyxiated in a short time.''[44]

Having performed the injection experiment described and observing the anticipated results, Bichat then turned to ''an experiment analogous to this one'' that relied on transfusion rather than injection. He connected the carotid arteries of two dogs by means of a silver tube so that the blood pumped by the heart of the first was pushed into the brain of the second. Then, asphyxiating the first animal, he saw the identical symptoms appearing in the second animal shortly after they were observed in the first.[45] Still another transfusion experiment was performed by Bichat later in his study of asphyxiation, to show the effects of black blood entering the arterial system in other parts of the body. This time the tube was attached to the crural artery of the recipient animal, with the result that the powers of motion and sensation in the dog's hind leg were lost when the donor animal was asphyxiated.[46]

Now the procedure followed in all these transfusion experiments—two by Bichat and three by Magendie—is clearly uniform. Both experimenters attempted to produce in the recipient animals the effects that they were inducing in the donor animals. Variations as to the particular effects in question or the particular organs of the body involved do not, of course, affect the isomorphism of the five experiments, as Table 4 illustrates.

VITALISM AND EXPERIMENTATION. As we have seen, for every experiment in Magendie's 1809 memoir on absorption, a parallel experiment can be found in Bichat's work on respiration and asphyxiation. This parallelism is not a matter of isolation applications of the same manipulative operation (blood transfusion, injection of an isolated part, etc.), but extends to the entire design, execution, and interpretation of each experiment in relation to the question posed for it. There are, of course, points of divergence as well, such as the opposition between the results the two men obtained in each set of experiments, or between Magendie's ability to apply the procedure used on the intestine to some other anatomical part and Bichat's inability to do this. But all these differences arise from the particular chemical or anatomical ''materials'' involved in the experiments and have no effect on their formal structure. Thus we may conclude that at the level of experimental technique Bichat and Magendie shared the same methodology.[47]

Nevertheless, in spite of their common experimental technique Bichat and Magendie took opposing positions on the subject of venous absorption. The reason for this opposition at first seems simple enough: Magendie investigated the subject experimentally and Bichat did not. But in the light of the comparative study that we have just completed, we must ask why Bichat, who was, as we have seen, technically capable of carrying out every experiment in Magendie's memoir, failed to apply the experimental method to the study of absorption. Was it, as the conventional account would suggest, his vitalism that stood as an obstacle to experimental inquiry?

Claude Bernard, for example, characterized Bichat in this way:

Bichat was not a pure experimenter, and he wanted, as he says himself in the preface to his *Researches on Life and Death,* to ally the experimental method of Haller and Spallanzani with the broad, philosophical views of [the vitalist] Bordeu. But it must be said that in this perilous alliance the experimenter quickly succumbed, and if Bichat at first depended upon the facts provided by experiments, he no longer consulted them when, carried away by his love of systems [*son esprit de système*], he created the vital properties of sensible and insensible contraction, of exhalation, etc. At this moment the broad, philosophical views of Bordeu subdued and killed the experimental method of Haller.[48]

According to this view, then, Bichat's overall method of physiological research was to begin from experimental evidence but, after a certain point, to rely upon vitalistic theorizing without attempting further experiments. If this view is substantially correct, then we can easily see how Magendie's criticism of Bichat's system of vital properties could be said to have removed a conceptual obstacle that was blocking the development of a fully experimental physiology.

But how adequate is this view of Bichat's research methodology? In order to evaluate Bernard's characterization and to determine whether or not it was Bichat's vitalism that restricted his use of physiological experimentation, we must first consider the methodological background evoked by the names of Haller, Spallanzani, and Bordeu. This background was the debate, which occupied the center of methodological controversy in late-eighteenth-century physiology and medicine, over the relative merits of observation and experimentation; and it was in light of this debate that Bichat, at the end of the century, consciously developed his own research methodology.

METHODOLOGICAL BACKGROUND. From the middle of the eighteenth century the physicians of the medical school at Montpellier in France had maintained that observation was the sole reliable source of data about living creatures. It was considered the glory of the school that their vitalistic interpretation of the phenomena of life was based entirely upon observation and reasoning, without recourse either to groundless speculation or to inconclusive experimentation. The philosophical doctrine of Montpellier was disseminated among the medical community through the writings of Théophile de Bordeu (1722–76) and was given even wider exposure through the articles contributed to Diderot's *Encyclopédie* by such spokesmen as Jean-Jacques Ménuret de Chambaud (1733–1815).[49] During the same period, however, experimental researches into physiological processes were being carried out on living animals with some success by figures such as the Swiss physician Albrecht von

Haller (1708–77) and the Italian naturalist Lazzaro Spallanzani (1729–99).
The objections of the Montpellier school to physiological experimentation
were posed chiefly on theoretical grounds. "The name of *observer,*" wrote
Ménuret,

has been given to the physicist who is content to examine the phenomena just as nature
presents them to him; he differs from the *experimental* physicist who combines himself
[with nature] and who sees only the result of his own combinations. This latter one
never sees nature as it is in fact; he pretends by his labor to render nature more
accessible to the senses, to raise the mask which conceals it from our eyes, but often he
disfigures it and renders it unintelligible. Nature is always unveiled and bare for him
who has eyes—or it is covered only by a slight gauze which the eye and reflection
easily pierce—and the pretended mask exists only in the imagination, usually quite
limited, of the manipulator [*manouvrier*] of experiments.[50]

Having set out this general position in his article "Observateur," Ménuret
went on to apply it to various classes of the sciences in his subsequent article
on "Observation."

Observation and experimentation are the only ways we have [leading] to knowledge, . . . and there is no doubt that *observation*, even in the physics of brute bodies,
infinitely overshadows experimentation both in certitude and utility. . . .

In passing from the physics of brute bodies to that of organized bodies, we shall see
the rights of *experimentation* diminish and the empire and utility of observation ex-
pand. . . .

Finally, man, from whatever aspect one envisions him, is the least proper to be
subject to *experimentation;* he is the most appropriate, the most noble, and the most
interesting object of *observation*, and it is only by *observation* that one can make any
progress in the sciences regarding man; here experimentation is often worse than
useless.[51]

In response to all such criticisms Haller replied simply that the results of the
experiments that he related were found to be "constantly true."[52] And because they revealed "several truths contrary to the opinions generally received," Haller continued, "I was obliged to repeat and multiply my experiments, in order to convince the incredulous, by a number of authentic tes-
timonies, so to speak, and prevent my falling accidentally into any mistake;
for I am persuaded that the great source of error in physic has been owing to
physicians, at least a great part of them, making few or no experiments, and
substituting analogy instead of them."[53]

Thus Haller answered theoretical objections with the pragmatic justification
that his experiments had produced uniform results throughout repeated trials.
From those whose opinions were contradicted by his experiments, Haller
asked only that they "defer condemning me, till they have compared the
experiments upon which [my own] opinion is founded"[54]—experiments repeated as often as "a hundred times" with the same result.[55] And should

anyone wish to disprove those results, Haller insisted that his opponent "must bring [forward] experiments such as mine. . . . But," he continued, "no such experiments can be produced; nature is too constant, and I have seen her act too often to be deceived in this point."[56]

Ménuret did not attack Haller's experiments directly in his articles on observation, but another of the Montpellier contributors to the *Encyclop-édie* did. This attack was contained in the article on sensibility written by Henri Fouquet (1727–1806), who dismissed Haller's argument from uniform results with the statement that even "the best-executed experiments are insufficient to advance our knowledge in a matter [of inquiry] whose delicate objects are denatured or disappear beneath the hand which seeks to manipulate them [*les travailler*]."[57]

The theoretical basis for this methodological attack lay in the Montpellier vitalists' emphasis upon the spontaneity of life. especially those self-regulative processes of living bodies which, as physicians, they referred to as "the healing power of nature."[58] For them observation provided the only possible way to study vital phenomena because the intervention of the experimenter necessarily destroyed the spontaneity of life by "denaturing" it. Uniform experimental procedures could, of course, yield uniform results: but phenomena produced in this way would always be "quite different from those presented by nature."[59]

Haller's position, too, for all its appearance of pragmatism, was firmly embedded in a theortical base, as his invocation of "the constancy of nature" indicates. For only by assuming that the phenomena of living bodies are "constant" in just the same way as those of nonliving bodies—i.e., that they are not spontaneous but instead are determined by fixed laws—could Haller argue from the uniformity of his experimental results to the reliability of those results as sources of information about the natural phenomena of life.

Beneath the methodological debate on experimentation and observation, then, lay fundamentally different conceptions of the character of living phenomena. The opposition between these conceptions did not take the familiar form of mechanism *versus* vitalism, however; for Haller was no more willing than the Montpellier physicians to attempt a mechanical or physico-chemical explanation of life.[60] The contrast, rather, was between Haller's postulation of the determinacy of vital phenomena and the Montpellier school's insistence upon the spontaneity of life and the independence of its phenomena from any fixed law.

BICHAT ON EXPERIMENTATION. Our discussion, in the previous section, of the two opposing methodological positions taken by physiologists in the last half of the eighteenth century, should provide us with the background necessary for undertaking an analysis of Bichat's research methodology. For Bichat, whose brief career began at the very end of the century, regarded both of these positions as one-sided and unsatisfactory in themselves. Thus he consciously set out to create a new method of physiological research that would combine the best aspects of both of the previous approaches, setting as his goal "the art of allying the experimental method of Haller and Spallanzani with the broad, philosophical views of Bordeu."[61]

To begin our investigation of how Bichat sought to bring about this alliance, let us consider his position regarding "Experiments on Living Animals," as set forth in his 1798 lecture on the study of physiology. Here, after noting the belief of one group of researchers "that physiology can only advance by means of experiments while the others [in the school of Montpellier] believe that they are fruitless," Bichat asked, "From what does this difference of opinion arise?" His answer was that both factions had approached the problem too generally, the one side advocating experiments without considering their limitations and the other side condemning experiments without considering their merits. Bichat's own view of the matter was that "in some cases experiments are advantageous, and in others they are very uncertain."[62]

Uncertainty in experimentation, for example, was "noted above all when the experiments have the vital forces as their object."[63] These "vital forces," which will be discussed in greater depth in the second part of this study, were held to be the ultimate explanatory principles in physiology, both by experimentalists such as Haller and by the advocates of pure observation. Although subject to various interpretations, these forces were generally identified as "sensibility," which enabled living matter to respond to stimuli, and "irritability" (or "contractility" or "motility"), which accounted for contraction or motion in living matter.

The experimental study of these vital forces, wrote Bichat, was often inconclusive because the pain and distress caused by the very act of experimentation was capable of changing the nature of these forces. In support of this contention he cited the fact that conflicting results had been obtained from some of Haller's experiments on sensibility;[64] thus challenging the validity of some of his eminent predecessor's findings, but not necessarily his contention that experimental results, if uniform, are a reliable source of physiological data. Accordingly, Bichat's concluding note on the subject was one of caution rather than inflexible opposition, as he recommended "great restraint in making pronouncements about the vital forces based upon experiments."[65]

Following this *caveat* Bichat called attention to "a multitude of other circumstances in which experiments give us very certain notions."[66] And although multifarious, these circumstances had, nonetheless, a common aspect, to judge from the examples listed by Bichat; for each of the experiments he mentioned was intended to reveal the sequence of events that occur during the exercise of one of the principal functions of life, such as digestion, respiration, absorption, secretion, and nutrition. "In all these cases," wrote Bichat, now sounding very much like Haller, "the experiments are certain; invariable results are drawn from them; but," he continued, "they demand extreme precision."[67] As a means of assuring this high degree of precision, and consequently of obtaining invariable results whenever possible, Bichat suggested four "general rules" to guide the experimenter. These rules included (1) comparison of the experimental animal with a normal one as a means of control, (2) the elimination of accidental interferences, (3) the repetition of the procedure, and (4) the necessity of giving due consideration to the state of the animal before and during the experiment.[68]

THE "INSTABILITY" OF LIFE. Bichat's fourth rule for experimentation brings us to the most important aspect of his vitalism insofar as his research methodology is concerned: his doctrine of the "instability" or extreme variability of the vital forces.[69] We have already seen that he, like Haller, considered the uniformity of experimental results in physiology to be a proof that those results gave "very certain notions" about the phenomena of life. This attitude would seem to indicate a deterministic view of life. On the other hand, we have also seen Bichat caution that the act of experimentation can change the nature of the vital forces, thus vitiating the experimental results. This opinion is reminiscent of the Montpellier school's claim that experimentation denatured the spontaneity of life; but the resemblance is deceptive, because Bichat's doctrine of the instability of the vital forces was different in significant ways from the Montpellier doctrine of the spontaneity of life.

Bichat saw natural phenomena as dependent upon two sets of laws. The first set comprised the laws of inorganic bodies, such as laws of gravity and elasticity. "Organized bodies," he continued, "also obey these laws, but in addition they obey the vital laws: sensibility and motility. There is a struggle, a continual effort between the physical and organic laws; the first laws are unceasingly modified by the second ones."[70] One could appreciate the effect of this continual process of modification of the physical laws in living bodies by contrasting the uniformity of physical phenomena with the perpetual variations of organic phenomena. One sees, wrote Bichat, that the vital laws are

unceasingly variable in their intensity, their energy, [and] their development, [they] often pass swiftly from the lowest degree of prostration to the highest point of exaltation, [they] are by turns built up and weakened in the organs and take on a thousand different modifications under the influence of the slightest causes. Sleep, waking, exercise, rest, digestion, hunger, the passions, the action of bodies external to the animal, etc., all expose the vital laws to numerous revolutions at each instant. The others [i.e., the physical laws], on the contrary—fixed, invariable, constantly the same at all times—are the source of a series of phenomena which are always uniform.[71]

Because of the stability of the physical laws, Bichat wrote, all the physical sciences were in principle subject to mathematization. But when applied to organic phenomena,

mathematics can never offer general formulas. One calculates the return of a comet, the resistances of a fluid traversing an inert channel, the swiftness of a projectile, etc.; but to calculate with Borelli the force of a muscle, with Keill the swiftness of the blood, with Jurine, Lavoisier and others the quantity of air entering the lungs, is to build upon quicksand an edifice which is solid in itself, but which soon collapses for lack of a secure base.

This instability of the vital forces, this ability which they have of varying in degree [*en plus ou en moins*] at each instant, impresses upon all the vital phenomena a character of irregularity which distinguishes them from the remarkably uniform physical phenomena.[72]

Bichat's pronouncements on the instability or variability of the vital forces have generally been misunderstood because of a failure to note the distinction between *normal* and *pathological* variations. His remarks about the uncertainty of experiments upon the vital forces referred to pathological changes in those forces. His comments in the two passages just quoted above, however, referred only to normal quantitative changes (*en plus ou en moins*) in the vital forces accompanying various nonpathological states (sleep, waking, exercise, etc.). To ascertain the significance of these two types of variations in the vital forces and their effect upon Bichat's research methodology, we must examine each of them more closely.

NORMAL VARIATIONS. Bichat compared the normal variations of the vital forces in a healthy subject to oscillations about a fixed point, using the image of a pendulum swinging to either side of its position of rest.[73] Such quantitative variations posed no obstacle to physiological experimentation, but only to the mathematization of physiology, as can be seen in the following statement by Bichat concerning his experiment on the coloring of blood which we previously examined:

When I indicate, in these phenomena, the precise time required for the coloring [of the dog's blood] to take place, I shall say only what I have seen, without pretending that the duration of the phenomena is uniform in man, nor even that this duration would be constant in animals examined in the diverse epochs of sleep, digestion, exercise, rest, or the passions, if it were possible to repeat the experiments in these diverse epochs. In general it is, as I have said, to know little of the animal functions to wish to submit them to the least calculation, because their instability is extreme. The phenomena remain always the same, and that is what matters to us; but their variations in degree [*en plus ou en moins*] are innumerable.[74]

Intimately related to this position on mathematics was Bichat's critical attitude toward the application of physics and chemistry to physiology. This attitude was apparent in the passage quoted above in which Borelli, Keill, and others were named as having founded exact calculations on inexact bases. The same theme was recurrent throughout Bichat's 1798 lecture on the relationship of physics and chemistry to physiology, in which he declared that "since the vital laws can never be the object of calculation, it is evident that mathematics has almost no application to physiology."[75] But while he attacked the unwarranted extension of mathematical laws from the physical sciences to the phenomena of life without due regard for the variability of the vital forces, he nevertheless recognized the importance of physics and chemistry in several areas. In physics, for example, he singled out such mathematical laws as those of optics, acoustics, and the various classes of levers as being necessary to the study of sight, hearing, and muscular locomotion.[76] Similarly, he acknowledged the value of chemical investigations into such functions as respiration, digestion, and nutrition.[77]

We may conclude, then, that Bichat's doctrine of the normal, quantitative variations of the vital forces posed no obstacle to physiological experimentation. At the level of experimental technique its only effect was to deter him from attempting a mathematical treatment of his data; and here again his experimental technique was shared by Magendie, who also "has been blamed for neglecting measurement."[78] But at the more general level of research methodology, which prescribes whether or not a phenomenon is to be studied experimentally, Bichat's doctrine of normal variations had no effect whatever.

PATHOLOGICAL VARIATIONS. An important part of his theory of the vital forces, Bichat held, was "that every pathological phenomenon derives from their augmentation, their diminution, or their alteration."[79] If the augmentation or diminution of the vital force did not, in a given case, distort the usual phenomena beyond recognition, then the effect would be the same as that of the normal quantitative variations discussed in the previous section. In most pathological affections, however, the vital forces were qualitatively altered, either by crossing a quantitative threshold[80] or by a simple change in their nature. "Consider the innumerable phenomena of diseases," wrote Bichat. "It is impossible to relate them to the known laws of sensibility—not only to relate them to known laws but even to found new laws upon these phenomena; because they do not resemble each other, they are all different and are diversely modified in diverse parts and in diverse affections."[81]

Now on Bichat's theory every vivisectional experiment should induce some pathological changes in the animal's vital forces because it would cause a wound. However, it was only when such changes took the form of qualitative alterations affecting the part or function of the animal that was under study, that the experimental results were unreliable. And his theory gave no *a priori* criteria for determining whether such qualitative alterations would result from a particular experiment. Consequently he could only judge *a posteriori*, by the uniformity or nonuniformity of the phenomena in the course of repeated trials, whether a given experiment had pathologically affected the vital forces so as to vitiate the resulting data.

Thus the doctrine of the pathological variations of the vital forces had no effect upon Bichat's research methodology. It was not a practical principle that ruled out certain experiments in advance, but rather an interpretive principle that explained the appearance of nonuniform experimental results despite the precautions of his four "general rules." For example, in the *Traité des membranes*, as a sequel to the experiment on the intestinal loop, he reported that the infiltration of oxygen gas into the "cellular" [i.e., connective] tissues of cats and guinea pigs sometimes produced a reddening of the blood in the vessels traversing the affected area, while other times it did not. Thus, he wrote,

although many experiments have been repeated on this point, I cannot indicate any general result. It seems that the tonic [i.e., contractile] forces of the cellular tissue and of the walls of the vessels which creep here and there throughout this tissue, receive a quite varied influence from the contact of gases, and that according to the nature of this influence the fibres tighten up and contract more or less, rendering these parts more or less permeable, ... which undoubtedly determines the variations which I have observed.[82]

The tentativeness of Bichat's explanation in the above example should be noted; for his invocation of pathological variations, as in this case of "artificial emphysema," did not prevent him from coming back to a phenomenon thus explained and accounting for it by new experiments. He returned, for example, to Haller's experiments on sensibility and showed that the inconsistent results previously obtained by other researchers had arisen from their unsystematic use of different means of stimulation. Hence he concluded, "The contradictory results which these experiments ... have offered must undoubtedly be attributed to the insensibility of fibrous membranes to one mode of excitation and their sensibility to another mode."[83] And to his earlier, general recommendation of "great restraint in making pronouncements about the vital forces based upon experiments," he added a specific methodological precept: "One must never pronounce upon the insensibility of an organ without having exhausted on it every means of irritation."[84]

Finally, we must consider one area in which Bichat's doctrine of pathological variations did serve as an obstacle to experimentation; namely, the area of pathology itself. Here it disuaded him from attempting "to produce artificially, in species different from our own, diseases similar to those which afflict us."[85] However, this line of experimental inquiry was not pursued by

Magendie either and did not become an accepted part of physiological research until the time of Claude Bernard, so we need not consider it further.

We may conclude, then, that Bichat's doctrine of the "instability" or variability of the vital forces, in both its normal and its pathological aspects, did not affect his research methodology in such a way as to restrain his use of physiological experimentation, and therefore that this doctrine was not a theoretical obstacle to the establishment of the experimental method in physiology. In other respects, however, Bichat's vitalism was not significantly different from Magendie's,[86] which suggests that some other factor should be sought to account for Bichat's restricted use of experimentation in physiological research. A clue to the identity of this factor may be found in his 1798 lecture on the study of physiology, to which we now return.

BICHAT ON OBSERVATION. At the beginning of his lecture Bichat identified three "sources from which the facts [of physiology] must be drawn . . . : 1st, observation of healthy men [and animals]; 2nd, experiments upon living animals; 3rd, observations upon diseased [men and] animals."[87] Now this enumeration in itself is not remarkable, for Magendie referred to the same three sources of data in his textbook of physiology, when he spoke of verifying the facts he presented in it "either by observation upon the healthy or diseased subject, or by experiments upon living animals."[88] What is noteworthy, however, is the central role that observation played in Bichat's research methodology.

To begin with, we may point to a very revealing ambiguity in Bichat's use of the term "observation." On the one hand, as we have seen above, he meant by this term a particular source of information about nature, in contrast to experimentation. But, on the other hand, he also used the same term to refer to experience in general, in contrast to reasoning; thus it was under the heading "Observational Physiology" (as opposed to "Rational Physiology") that he enumerated and examined the three sources of physiological facts, including experimentation.[89] This terminological ambiguity marks a crucial feature of Bichat's research methodology that will allow us to distinguish it, provisionally at least, from the research methodologies followed by the Montpellier physicians, by Haller and by Magendie.

Unlike the Montpellier physicians, Bichat did not place simple observation (observation in the narrow sense) and experimentation in radically different epistemological categories. For him, experiments were merely one other form of "observation" (in the general sense of "experience")—a form demanding "extreme precision" when applied in physiology, but nevertheless capable of providing information about nature which was as reliable as that obtained from simple observation. Bichat's epistemology, then, offered no grounds for the *a priori* rejection of experimental data as artefacts unrelated to natural processes, just as his metaphysics contained no commitment to the absolute spontaneity of life.

Bichat's use of the term "observation" to designate experience in general, however, is symptomatic of the fact that, unlike Haller and Magendie, he assigned priority to simple observation as a means of acquiring physiological data.[90] For although experimentation could, in his eyes, be as reliable as simple observation in providing specific factual information, it was nevertheless not a fruitful source of "broad, philosophical views"—of those general concepts regarding life and its phenomena that provided an integrative framework for the individual facts disclosed by experiments.

Attaining a broad, philosophical view of life meant, for Bichat, beginning one's research not with experiments upon particular physiological processes, such as sensation or contraction, but with the observation of life-phenomena as a whole. Haller's failure to carry out his experiments within a sufficiently general context was, in Bichat's eyes, one of the factors that led him to erroneous conclusions. "Haller occupied himself above all with sensibility and irritability; but in limiting the first to the nervous system and the second to the muscular system, this great man did not consider these properties from the true point of view at all; he made almost isolated properties of them."[91] The basis of Bichat's research methodology was observation; only when the practical limits of observation had been reached—when the naturally occurring phenomena were too complex, minute or scarce to be studied by simple observation—did he take up experimentation to push his analysis further. This order of priority is strikingly illustrated in the organization of his *Recherches physiologiques sur la vie et la mort*.

Bichat began his work with the famous observational definition of life as "the totality of the functions which resist death."[92] This totality he then divided by observation, "the simplest and most natural" method, into "two great classes of functions: the one external and the other internal."[93] These two classes of functions (designated in the *Recherches physiologiques* as the "animal" and "organic" lives, respectively) were further subdivided, again on the basis of observation.

It is this method that reveals to us that the exterior life is composed: 1st, of the action of the senses, of sensations; 2nd, of perception by the brain; 3rd, of the will and the judgement; 4th, of locomotion.

It is this method which reveals to us a double movement in the interior life—[one] of composition by means of the nutrients and [one] of decomposition by means of the excrements, perspiration, insensible transpiration, etc.[94]

Having established these preliminary divisions, Bichat devoted the rest of the first part of his book ("Recherches physiologiques sur la vie") to an examination of the differences between animal life and organic life in respect to the forms of their organs; the mode of action of their organs; the duration of their actions; their relation to habits; their relation to the intellect and emotions; their vital forces; their origin and development; and, finally, their natural termination. Throughout this entire study Bichat relied almost completely upon observation—primarily upon the observation of healthy subjects and secondarily upon pathological observation.[95] In one paragraph only did he cite experiments, and there he merely reported the results of experiments that he described elsewhere.[96]

In the second part of his book ("Recherches physiologiques sur la mort") Bichat studied the question, which had been raised by the conclusion of the first part of his work, regarding the difference between the phenomena of natural death and those of sudden death.[97] Here he relied heavily upon experiments, many of which were very elaborate, in his investigation of the sequences of phenomena by which death occurs when one of the three principal organs—the brain, the heart, or the lungs—ceases to function. But even in this part of his work his experiments were extensively supplemented by pathological observations and carried out entirely within the conceptual framework established in the first part of the book on the basis of observation.

The order of priority in Bichat's research methodology, then, which underlay his *Recherches physiologiques* as a whole, was as follows: (1) observation of the normal subject, (2) pathological observation, (3) experimentation. And this same order was adhered to in the physiological sections of his other works, from his "Mémoire sur la membrane synoviale" of 1799,[98] his first nonsurgical publication, to his posthumous *Anatomie descriptive*.

The privileged status of observation in Bichat's methodology was highlighted by the position that he took on the theoretical limitations to this means of research. Indeed, the only theoretical limits that he recognized for physiological observation were those set by anatomical observation. In order for the observation of healthy subjects to be effective, he insisted that the observer must have detailed knowledge of the anatomical substrate of the physiological phenomena. "Although the physicians of Montpellier regarded the science [of physiology] in a philosophical manner" wrote Bichat, "they would have caused it to make more progress if they had known more anatomy—Haller caused it to make such great progress only because of this''[99] In addition, he held that the same functions must be observed in animals of different anatomical composition for comparison.[100] Finally, in the observation of pathological phenomena, the only diseases that he thought could "cast much light on physiology" were those that disturbed the anatomical organization of the patient, such as tumors, cataracts, etc.[101] These "organic diseases" functioned for Bichat in the manner of natural experiments, in that they altered particular anatomical parts without the need for vivisection.

So as we see, there were no theoretical limits imposed by Bichat's epistemology that would require him to turn from observation to experimentation for physiological data. Only practical limitations on observation led him to perform experiments.[102] And it was this use of experimentation as an extension of observation, alien though it was to the epistemology of the Montepellier school, which prevented Bichat the brilliant experimenter from becoming a true experimentalist.

RESEARCH PROBLEMATICS. In Bichat's research methodology, observation of the normal subject established the main divisions and as many subordinate ones as possible. These divisions were then confirmed and sometimes extended by means of pathological observations. Finally, experiments were employed to systematize and further confirm the observational data already collected, and to resolve questions that had been raised but left unanswered by observation. However, it was not the function of these experiments to raise new questions for research or to test the general analytical framework established by observation.

Bichat's research methodology, then, was governed by a problematic of observation; that is, observation not only played the major role in the resolution of problems but also definied what *were* and, equally importantly, what *were not* the problems that needed to be resolved. For Bichat the progress of physiology depended upon starting with a global conception of life derived from observation, a conception which was increasingly refined—but never fundamentally challenged—by a series of divisions or analyses. These analyses, based upon observation where possible and experimentation where necessary, served to fill in more and more detail, thus enriching—but also subtly confirming—the initial conception of life with which the study began.

Magendie's research methodology, on the contrary, was governed by a problematic of experimentation. He approached physiology as a science to be built up bit by bit, from the bottom as it were, beginning with the data of individual experiments. At the very outset of his career he was already insisting that "most physiological facts need to be verified by new experiments";[103] and in later years "his work more and more took on the character of a mere conglomeration of experimental results."[104] According to Claude Bernard, "M. Magendie, who was the pure experimenter *par excellence*, always wished to hear only of the brute and isolated experimental result, without the intervention of any systematic idea either as point of departure or as consequence."[105] The experiments from which these results were obtained were rarely more sophisticated in design or execution than those of Bichat, but their function within Magendie's research methodology was entirely different.

This difference may be illustrated by returning once again to the subject of venous absorption. In Magendie's case, research on this subject began, as we have seen, with a series of experiments to determine how the poison *upas tieuté* caused the death of its victims. But the results of these first experiments, which showed that the immediate cause of death was asphyxiation, served not only to answer the original question but also to raise new questions: "Is the upas really absorbed?" and "Does the upas penetrate into the circulatory system?" and finally, "What part of the nervous system does it act upon?"[106] Each of these three questions was resolved experimentally, but the data from these experiments suggested a further question: "Does the poison, which acts so quickly when injected into a muscle, reach the bloodstream through the lymphatic system?" And it was to investigate this question that Magendie carried out a new series of experiments resulting in his demonstration of venous absorption.

Bichat's point of departure, on the other hand, was the observation that the lymphatic system was the agent of absorption for chyle and certain other substances. These observed instances Bichat took as representative of all absorption, so that the only question left to be resolved was "whether the absorbents arise from [any given part of the body, and] consequently whether absorption is observed there."[107] Thus Bichat's experiments on "venous absorption" were precisely the opposite in intention from Magendie's. Testing the opinion that "the absorbents arise immediately from the veins and arteries," Bichat experimented to determine whether a substance (the serous portion of the blood) passed from the bloodstream into the lymphatic system;[108] whereas, Magendie experimented to determine whether a substance (*upas*) passed through the lymphatic system into the bloodstream.

The methodological opposition between Bichat and Magendie, then, originated not at the level of experimental techniques (a crude technique *versus* a sophisticated one), nor at the level of metaphysical conceptions of life (vitalism *versus* mechanism, or spontaneity *versus* determinism), but at the level of research problematics (a problematic of observation *versus* a problematic of experimentation). On the other hand, it is important to note that in spite of the *apparent* difference between them, the research methodologies of Bichat, Haller, and the Montpellier physicians all nevertheless shared the same problematic of observation. All three of these methodologies were variations constructed according to the same set of rules, whereas Magendie's methodology arose from a different set of rules altogether.

We have already shown that Bichat's research methodology consisted of starting with observation of the whole, progressive analysis by means of observation to the practical limit of that method, and, finally, further analysis by means of experiments. This methodology we may schematically represent as follows:

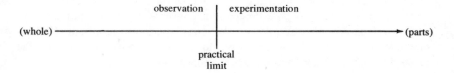

Similarly, the Montpellier methodology commenced with observation of the whole and progressively analyzed the phenomena to the limit of observation. But at this point the Montpellier physicians saw an epistemological barrier to further analysis. Since, for them, experiments on living bodies produced only "denatured" phenomena, the limit of observation was at the same time the limit of reliable information about life. Because of the obstacle presented by this concept of the spontaneity of life, the physiology of the Montpellier school reached an absolute epistemological limit (the point at which the pursuit of knowledge in a given area had to halt), whereas Bichat's physiology recognized only a practical limit (the point at which one form of practice—observation—had to be replaced by another form—experimentation—directed toward the same goal). We may thus represent the Montpellier methodology as follows:

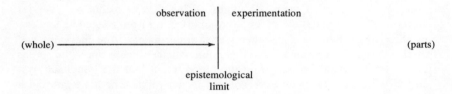

Finally, Haller's methodology also functioned within the same problematic of observation, for his experimental researches began with a preexisting set of concepts, such as "sensibility" and "irritability," which previous generations of physicians had established on the basis of careful observation of the phenomena of life. Haller's experiments were not intended to raise new questions for physiological research, but only to define more clearly these historically-given "vital properties" and to systematize the knowledge of their distribution among the various parts of the body by means of uniform tests.[109] Haller, like Bichat, experimented entirely within the limited framework provided by concepts derived from observation; but unlike Bichat, he did not attempt to present his own exhaustive observational account of these concepts before turning to experiments. Thus, in Haller's methodology, the limit set between observation and experimentation served as the *terminus a quo* of the latter procedure but not as the *terminus ad quem* of the former: it was a limit to the conceptual grounding that Haller sought for his experiments. He did not start from observations of life-phenomena as a whole in order to offer a systematic foundation for the concepts on which these experiments depended; instead, he simply accepted such concepts as products of the historical development of physiology. We may therefore represent Haller's methodology in the following way, to show its relationship with the methodologies of Bichat and the Montpellier school:

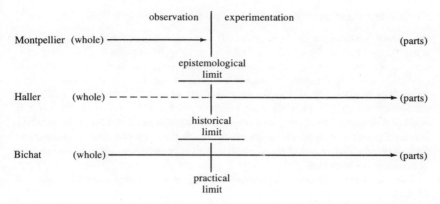

We see, then, how it was possible for Bichat to ally the methods of Bordeu and Haller: since they both operated within the problematic of observation Bichat could use each one to supplement and extend the other within that same problematic. Where the Hallerian method silently passed over the foundations of its historically-given interpretation of life, Bichat applied the method of Montpellier to provide a philosophical basis for that interpretation (e.g., part I of the *Recherches physiologiques*); where the method of Montpellier halted before an epistemological barrier, Bichat saw only a practical limit and applied the method of Haller (e.g., part II of the *Recherches physiologiques*). Thus we cannot accept Claude Bernard's judgment that Bichat's methodology was a "perilous alliance" of mutually incompatible methods in which "the broad philosophical views of Bordeu subdued and killed the experimental method of Haller."[110] In fact, the methods were not only compatible, but were complementary.

The fundamental methodological incompatibility was not between the methods of Bordeu and Haller or between those of Haller and Bichat. The fundamental methodological incompatibility was, rather, between the research problematic of observation shared by Bichat, Haller, and Bordeu, and the research problematic of experimentation introduced into physiology by Magendie. Thus far, however, we have only been able to identify and describe these research problematics. In the second part of our study, after a consideration of the question of physiological explanation, we shall be able to relate these research problematics to their underlying foundations as well.

Part II: Explanation

INTRODUCTION. In the preface to his physiology textbook of 1816–17, Magendie distinguished two forms in which a natural science might exist, the "systematic" and the "theoretical." "Under the systematic form," he wrote,

the science is founded upon some gratuitous suppositions, some principles established *a priori*, to which known facts are attached so as to be explained. If a new fact is discovered, which does not accord with the fundamental principle, this [principle] is modified till it furnishes an explanation which gives satisfaction: if the learned give themselves up to the labour of experiment, it is always with the intention of confirming the system which has been adopted: every thing that can tend to overthrow it is neglected or unperceived; they seek after what ought to be, not what is; in short the synthetic course is completely followed, in which they descend from hypotheses to facts, without rising to any of the general consequences which ought to be had in view in the inquiries after truth.

When this form is observed, it is almost impossible for a natural science to make real progress.

The theoretic form of natural science is diametrically opposite to this. Facts, and facts alone, constitute the foundation of the science, under this form: the learned endeavour to verify them, and to multiply them as much as possible, and afterwards study the relations of the different phenomena, and the laws to which they are subject. When they give themselves up to experimental researches, it is with the view of augmenting the number of ascertained facts, or to discover their reciprocal relation; in a word, the analytical course is followed, which alone can lead to truth. By following this method, the sciences increase, if not rapidly, at least surely, and we may hope to see them approach perfection.[111]

As Owsei Temkin has remarked in his discussion of the paragraphs just quoted, "These words might as well have been written 20 years before."[112] Both the position taken by Magendie and the language in which he expressed it were quite in keeping with the philosophical tradition of the late-eighteenth century, and particularly with the French representative of that tradition known as *idéologie*.[113] Bichat, who has sometimes been included among the *idéologues,* would certainly have subscribed to Magendie's formulation in every particular.

Nevertheless, Magendie's preface went on to claim that "physiology, so important a branch of natural knowledge, has hitherto preserved its systematic form," and that consequently it "is still in its infancy."[114] Such an assertion, concluded Temkin, coming as it did fourteen years after the death of Bichat, "reveals the point where Magendie had developed beyond the tradition of the idéologues."[115] In Magendie's eyes Bichat's physiology was systematic and synthetic, while in Bichat's own eyes it was theoretic and analytic.

Clearly, some fundamental change had taken place in physiology since the death of Bichat—a change that allowed Magendie, "applying the same philosophical arguments under different circumstances,"[116] to attack Bichat's research methodology on precisely the grounds that Bichat considered it most secure and well-founded. It was this change, the nature of which we shall examine here in the second part of of our study, that underlay not only the opposition between Bichat's problematic of observation and Magendie's problematic of experimentation but the birth of modern physiology as well.

MAGENDIE'S MANIFESTO OF 1809. At the core of Magendie's criticism of the physiological method of his predecessors, was his dissatisfaction with the generally accepted manner of explaining the phenomena of life. Even "in the best works," he wrote in 1816, "we find [physiology] founded upon mere suppositions, to which everyone attaches at pleasure the numerous phenomena of life, thinking that he is explaining them satisfactorily."[117] Seven years earlier Magendie had published a paper entirely devoted to this question of physiological explanation, entitled "Quelques idées générales sur les phénomènes particuliers aux corps vivans."[118] Here, in what has been called "the manifesto of the new physiology,"[119] he set out the theoretical position to which he adhered throughout his career. It is on the basis of this paper, then, that we shall investigate the change that set his physiology apart from all previous work in that field.

Magendie opened his essay with a thoroughly traditional statement on the logical form of a developed science: "The character of a certain and perfected science is that it has as its base only a small number of principles to which a great number of facts are easily connected." The physical sciences, he continued, such as "chemistry, physics and above all astronomy," exhibit this logical form; but physiology cannot lay claim to such a distinction, in spite of the impressive achievements of the last fifty years—that is, since about the time of Haller.[120] To remedy this deficiency, Magendie said that he hoped to set physiology on the same path as that which the physical sciences were following, by proving two points: (1) that the present manner of regarding the phenomena proper to living bodies is unsound in several respects; and (2) that these phenomena can all be explained in the same manner.[121]

On the first of these points, Magendie criticized "the physiologists"—he did not single out any individual in particular—for invoking a number of special, vital "principles," "properties," "powers," or "forces" to explain the phenomena of life. These explanatory entities—chiefly sensibility and contractibility—were briefly mentioned in the first part of this study, in connection with Bichat's statement on "the uncertainty of experiments." But before we can adequately discuss Magendie's attack on the use of such explanatory principles we must consider them in some detail. In doing so we shall use Bichat's system as our primary illustration and then present other systems more briefly by way of comparison.

BICHAT'S SYSTEM OF VITAL PROPERTIES. For Bichat, the animal and organic lives each had its own characteristic forms of sensibility and contractility.[122] He thus subdivided these two properties according to their modes of manifestation in the two lives. "Animal sensibility" was the faculty of receiving an impression and of relating it to the common sensory center of the brain; hence its exercise was always accompanied by conscious perception. "Animal contractility" was likewise dependent upon the brain, in that its exercise was subject to the commands of the will. Since animal contractility was exercised voluntarily, it did not uniformly follow upon the exercise of animal sensibility, nor was its intensity related to the intensity of the sensations perceived by the subject.

"Organic sensibility," on the other hand, was the faculty of receiving an impression and relating it only to a local ganglionic center; thus it represented a mode of unperceived sensation known only by its effects. These effects, in turn, were dependent upon "organic contractility," a faculty of contraction that was independent of the will and always exercised in proportion to the degree of organic sensation that provoked it. In some cases of organic contractility, such as the contraction of the involuntary muscles, the phenomenon itself was evident to the observer; but in other cases, such as the motions within the glands causing secretions, it was either too minute or too slow to be observed. Therefore, Bichat divided this property into two kinds, which he called "sensible organic contractility" and "insensible organic contractility." He considered it impossible, however, to draw a definite line of demarcation between these two subdivisions of organic contractility; so he referred to them merely as varieties of organic contractility rather than as separate vital properties.

Although organic contractility could never be converted into animal contractility (since the involuntary movements of the body were thought by Bichat to be free of all control by the will), the same was not true of organic and animal sensibility. Bichat noted cases in which a part endowed only with organic sensibility became painful as a result of inflammation and concluded that these two types of sensibility differed only in degree. Nevertheless, he continued to treat them as separate vital properties because the difference between them was set by nature rather than by the limitations of the observer; that is, as organic sensibility was increased in degree it changed abruptly, rather than continuously, into animal sensibility, indicating the existence of a natural threshold between the two forms.

Having set out these details, we may summarize Bichat's system of the vital properties by means of the following chart, in which the vertical scale (from bottom to top) represents the degree of intensity of the properties and the horizontal scale (from left to right) represents the sequence in which the phenomena take place (Fig. 2).

Bichat held that each of the tissues of the body, of which he distinguished twenty-one kinds in his *Anatomie générale*, was endowed with some or all of these vital properties, each in a characteristic degree.[123] At the bare

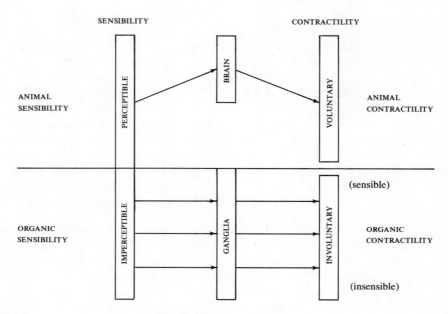

Fig. 2. Bichat's system of vital properties

minimum, each living tissue required organic sensibility and insensibile organic contractility in order to maintain its existence, for these properties enabled it to appropriate nutriment from the bloodstream and to expel waste materials. By organic sensibility each tissue became sensible of the presence of waste materials within it and of nutriments surrounding it in the blood; then by insensible organic contractility it rejected those wastes and selected from the bloodstream the nutriments proper to it, leaving all others.[124]

In addition to these two basic properties, however, most tissues were endowed with more specialized properties: the tissue of the heart—or stomach—muscle, for example, with sensible organic contractility; that of the skin with animal sensibility; that of the voluntary muscles with animal contractility; etc. And it was one of the major tasks that Bichat undertook in his *Anatomie générale* to determine precisely the degree to which each of these vital properties could be found in each of the twenty-one bodily tissues.[125]

OTHER SYSTEMS OF VITAL PROPERTIES. Although Bichat's system of vital properties attained great prominence in France in the years after his death, it was by no means the only such system available at the time. Nevertheless, Claude Bernard, in his eulogy of Magendie, described the 1809 paper as "a critique of the vital properties of Bichat";[126] and nearly every subsequent commentator has accepted this judgment. The consensus has thus been that Magendie's strictures were directed "against Bichat, or Bichat's follow-ers."[127] Now it is true that Magendie's criticisms, which we shall examine hereafter, applied to the system set out by Bichat in the *Recherches physiologiques* and *Anatomie générale;* and it is also true that Magendie mentioned Bichat by name in his text.[128] However, Magendie also referred, directly or indirectly, to at least four other French physiologists—Paul-Joseph Barthez (1734–1806), François Chaussier (1746–1828), Charles-Louis Dumas (1765–1813), and Balthasar-Anthelme Richerand (1779–1840)—none of whom could properly be characterized as a follower of Bichat. We shall therefore briefly describe the systems of vital properties found in the works of these four physiologists and attempt to show the common ground that they all shared with the system of Bichat, before passing on to Magendie's critique of the use of vital properties as explanatory entities.

1. *Barthez,* who considered himself the successor to the mantle of Bordeu at Montpellier, first published his *Nouveaux éléments de la science de l'homme* in 1778, and he produced a second, expanded edition of this work in 1806. According to Barthez, the phenomena of life resulted from a "vital principle" that manifested itself in the form of two kinds of "forces". The first group of forces he called "motive forces,"[129] which he distinguished into "muscular forces" (found in the muscular fibers and characterized by rapid motion),[130] "tonic forces" (found everywhere in the body and charac-terized by slow motion),[131] and "the force of fixed situation" (the force that prevented the fibers from tearing apart under tension).[132] The second group of forces Barthez named "sensitive forces";[133] these, he said, were manifested as "local sensibility" (not consciously perceived, present in all parts, inde-pendent of the nerves) and "general sensibility" (consciously perceived, not present in all parts, dependent upon the nervous system).[134]

2. *Chaussier* was professor of anatomy and physiology at the Paris medical school after the revolution, and he prepared his *Table synoptique des prop-riétés characteristiques et des principaux phénomènes de la force vitale* as a teaching aid for use with his lectures. The first edition of this folio-sized sheet carried no date, but a second edition appeared in the year IX (1800–01). In his *Table synoptique* Chaussier identified the properties of the "vital force" as "motility" (the faculty of movement), "sensibility" (the faculty of feeling), and "caloricity" (the faculty of producing heat). He noted that sensibility, present in all parts of all living beings, was exercised in different ways in the various organs, but he did not assign special names to these manifestations. Motility, however, Chaussier divided into "tonicity" (which he also called "vital tension, fibrillary contractility, or tonic force") and "myotility" (or, alternatively, "Hallerian irritability, or muscular con-

tractility"). The first of these two types of motility was that of the simple fibers, while the second was found only in the muscles.[135]

3. *Dumas,* another representative of the Montpellier school, distinguished four "physiological forces or powers." "I designate these four powers," he wrote in his *Principes de physiologie* of 1801, "by the arbitrary and conventional names of *sensitive force, contractile force, assimilative force,* and *force of vital resistance*. The first embraces the properties which cause feeling, the second those which produce movement, the third those which bring about nutrition, and finally the last comprehends those which maintain the animal body or its parts in a permanent and fixed situation."[136] The faculty of feeling, Dumas continued, was common to all parts of the body; but it was exercised in two forms: "it is obscure, *latent* and dull in certain parts; evident, manifest, appreciable in others."[137] Similarly, all parts of the body enjoyed the power of movement, according to him; but here again in two forms: "the one continual, obscure, hidden, which only becomes apparent when it receives an extraordinary increase; the other manifest, visible, which shows itself only by intervals, sometimes under the impression of a stimulus and sometimes under the orders of the will."[138] Unlike the physiologists whose systems we have previously studied, Dumas did not think that nutrition could be accounted for by means of sensibility and contractility, "for assimilation in no way resembles sensations or contractions."[139] It would be more reasonable, he held, to regard sensibility and contractility as effects of the assimilative force, since the organs are formed by nutrition and develop their sensible and contractile powers during that process.[140] The remaining force identified by Dumas, the force of vital resistance, corresponded to Barthez's force of fixed situation, except that Dumas ranked it as a force independent of sensibility and contractility, while Barthez considered it simply as a particular type of motive force.[141]

4. *Richerand,* the last physiologist whom we shall consider, was a younger colleague of Bichat's in Paris who first published his *Nouveaux éléments de physiologie* in 1801. In this textbook Richerand recognized only two vital properties, sensibility and contractility, each of which existed under "two great modifications." The two forms of sensibility he called "*percevant sensibility*" ("with consciousness of the impressions, or *perceptibility:* it requires a particular apparatus [of sensory organs]") and "*latent or vegetative sensibility*" ("without consciousness of the impressions, or *general sensibility,* and common to all that has life: it has no special organ and is found universally in all living parts, animal or vegetable"). Contractility was divided by Richerand into voluntary and involuntary contractility, and this latter form subdivided according to whether it could be observed or not; thus yielding the following types:

> *Voluntary and sensible* [*contractility*], subordinated to *perceptibility*.
> *Involuntary and insensible* [*contractility*[, corresponding to general and
> latent sensibility.
> *Involuntary and sensible* [*contractility*].[142]

In all these divisons Richerand's system resembled Bichat's; nevertheless, the similarity between these two particular systems of vital properties should not be overemphasized. For if we leave aside Barthez's force of fixed situation, Chaussier's caloricity, and Dumas' forces of assimilation and vital resistance, we find that the systems of these three physiologist fundamentally agreed with those of Bichat and Richerand. This agreement can be summarized in Table 5.

MAGENDIE'S CRITIQUE OF VITAL PROPERTIES. Now that we have surveyed the various systems of vital properties devised by physiologists whose works were prominent in the early years of the nineteenth century,[143] we may turn to

TABLE 5
Comparison of Systems of Vital Properties

	I. General term for the first vital property	*I–A. Term for this property when perceptible*	*I–B. Term for this property when imperceptible*
BICHAT	SENSIBILITY	Animal sensibility	Organic sensibility
RICHERAND	SENSIBILITY	Perceptibility, or percevant sensibility	Latent, vegetative, general sensibility
BARTHEZ	SENSITIVE FORCES	General sensibility	Local sensibility
DUMAS	SENSITIVE FORCES	Evident, manifest, appreciable sensation	Obscure, latent, dull sensation
CHAUSSIER	SENSIBILITY	(not further subdivided)	

	II. General term for the second vital property	*II–A. Term for this property when observable*		*II–B. Term for this property when unobservable (and involuntary)*
		II–A–1. Voluntary	*II–A–2. Involuntary*	
BICHAT	CONTRACTILITY	Animal contractility	Sensible organic contractility	Insensible organic contractility
RICHERAND	CONTRACTILITY	Voluntary and sensible contractility	Involuntary and sensible contractility	Involuntary and insensible contractility
BARTHEZ	MOTIVE FORCES	Muscular forces		Tonic forces
DUMAS	CONTRACTILE FORCES	Manifest, visible contraction		Continual, obscure, hidden contraction
CHAUSSIER	MOTILITY	Myotility, Hallerian irritability, or muscular contractility		Tonicity, vital tension, fibrillary contractility, or tonic force

Magendie's criticisms of that approach to physiological explanation. These criticisms we shall consider under four headings.

1. *Generality*. While some of the vital properties were said to be inherent in all parts of all living organisms and were thus general properties of life, others were restricted to certain parts of certain classes of organisms. For example, the properties of "organic sensibility" and "insensible organic contractility," or their equivalents, were attributed to all parts of all living organisms and were supposed by most physiologists to be responsible for the nutrition of each of those parts. On the other hand, only certain parts of animals—the voluntary muscles—were said to be endowed with the property of "animal contractility." But, Magendie argued, "a vital property ought to characterize life everywhere that the vital force has any influence; it ought to be common to all living bodies in the same way that extension, divisibility, impenetrability and mobility are the general properties of all bodies."[144] Thus he concluded that properties that were limited to particular parts of bodies, or to particular phenomena only, ought not to be admitted. Among such particular properties he included "sensible organic contractility," "animal sensibility," and "animal contractility,"[145] as well as "an assimilative force, a force of fixed situation, a force of vital resistance, etc."[146]

2. *Positivity*. Even though the properties of "organic sensibility" and "insensible organic contractility" were not affected by the first criticism, because they were attributed to all parts of all organisms, they were nevertheless wholly imperceptible and thus purely hypothetical. "These terms," wrote Magendie, ". . . designate no appreciable phenomena but only pure suppositions, simple manners of conceiving."[147] Hence, he reasoned, they offered no real explanation and provided no positive knowledge of the phenomena.[148]

3. *Vital Action*. The property of "sensible organic contractility," in addition to being a particular rather than a general property, was also subject to attack from another point of view. The contractions of the involuntary muscles, such as those of the heart or stomach, ought not to be attributed to a special property, said Magendie, because they were simply the products of the "action" of the muscles in question, just as bile and urine were the products of the "action" of the liver and kidneys.[149] This concept of "action" will be made clearer in the following section when we consider Magendie's proposals for a new explanatory system in physiology.

4. *Function*. Like "sensible organic contractility," the properties of "animal sensibility" and "animal contractility" were criticized by Magendie on other grounds in addition to those of generality. "I am prepared to admit, for the moment," he wrote, "that a vital property need not be common to all living bodies; but it ought, at least, to reside uniquely in the part in which it is supposed to exist."[150] But animal sensibility, he continued, was not really a property of the sense-organ, nor of the nerve, nor of the brain, because its

exercise required the cooperation of all three of these organs. "If one of these organs is lacking, or if it is slightly altered, there is no animal sensibility at all."[151] For Magendie, then, "animal sensibility" was not a vital property but rather a "function"—the result of the combined "actions" of the sense-organs, the nerves and the brain.[152] Similarly, he considered "animal contractility" to be a "function" resulting from the combined "actions" of the brain, the nerves and the voluntary muscles.[153]

MAGENDIE'S EXPLANATORY SYSTEM. The second aim of Magendie's paper, it will be recalled, was to show that all the phenomena of life could be explained in the same way. To accomplish this task, he pointed out that all these phenomena could be reduced to two principal characteristics of living organisms: nutrition and action.[154]

By "nutrition" Magendie meant the assimilation of nutritive matter by each living "molecule" of an organism, and the excretion by these molecules of matter no longer suitable to make up part of their composition. The double motion of composition and decomposition resulting in nutrition, he wrote, "is not perceptible to our senses, and consequently its mode of action is entirely unknown to us; nevertheless, since we definitely see matter displaced, it becomes certain for us that there has been movement."[155]

As to the cause of nutrition, Magendie conceded that

No analogy, not even a probable one, has yet been found between the play of ordinary chemical affinities and the nutritive movement; that is why this movement has always been considered—and still is today—as dependent upon a particular cause which, like planetary and molecular attraction, is unknown in its nature but manifest in its effects. This particular cause has received many denominations, but the best which has been given is that of *vital force*. Up to this point our reasoning is perfect. . . .[156]

But the physiologists, he continued, persist in attempting to explain the manner in which "each molecule animated by the vital force acts in order to produce this nutritive movement. . . ."[157] This they do by the supposition of the properties known as "organic sensibility" and "insensible organic contractility." These properties, as we have seen, Magendie considered wholly gratuitous; nevertheless he consented to accept them as a provisional hypothesis. "But," he warned, "the savant who has some idea of the means necessary for experimenting and for advancing the science ought not to delude himself about the true value of these expressions. What would be worth much more still than all these reasonings would be to perform experiments with a view to finding the general laws of the vital force."[158]

The second general characteristic of life Magendie called "action." By this term he meant the particular activities exhibited by each of the organs: contraction in the muscles, production of bile in the liver, and so on. Like nutrition, he considered action to be the result of an intestine motion arising from the same vital force as that causing the nutritive movement.[159] But whereas nutrition was a motion of decomposition and recomposition occurring within each living molecule individually, action was the motion of organized groups of these molecules: "it seems," wrote Magendie, "to be the result of an intestine movement which takes place among the living molecules of the acting organ."[160]

With this conception of nutrition and action, Magendie had established the foundation of the second aim of his paper. For, as he put it, "If it were possible at this time to prove that all the phenomena of organized bodies can be related to nutrition or action, these phenomena could be regarded as produced by the same force, and they would be explained naturally in the same manner."[161] And in the balance of his paper he attempted to show that all the phenomena hitherto explained by the "particular" vital properties could be reduced to actions that the organs performed singly or, in the case of functions, in groups. In relying on the vital properties, he wrote, "the physiologists have based their science upon an unsteady scaffolding. . . . But by bringing all the phenomena proper to living bodies into connection with nutrition and action. . . . we would permit that scaffolding to collapse of its own weight."[162]

What Magendie proposed, then, was an interpretation of the phenomena of life based upon a unique vital force that was responsible both for the changing chemical composition of each living molecule (nutrition) and for the changing spatial relationships between these molecules (action). The molecular movements of these two principal phenomena could, if one wished, "be easily explained by organic sensibility and insensible [organic] contractility."[163] But Magendie insisted that these hypothetical properties added nothing positive to the science of life, and in 1816 he rejected them outright "as useless and dangerous suppositions."[164]

Now the molecular motions of nutrition and action could not be the objects of direct scientific study, since they were wholly imperceptible. Therefore Magendie concuded his paper by advising his colleagues "to commence the study of physiology at the instant when the phenomena of living bodies become appreciable to our senses," and to spend their time "in performing experiments and in describing important phenomena with exactitude."[165]

Having seen Magendie's criticism of his predecessors in physiology and his own proposals for the reform of that science, we may now ask what fundamental change the "manifesto" of 1809 represented. Certainly the call for experimentation was not new with him. Although the Montpellier physiologists—Barthez and Dumas—eschewed experimentation, the representatives of the Paris school—Bichat, Chaussier, and Richerand—encouraged, performed, and relied upon experiments to provide them with physiological data.[166] It was not the lack of experiments but the explanatory framework within which they had been carried out that led Magendie to the belief that "most physiological facts need to be verified by new experiments, and that this is the sole means of rescuing the physics of living bodies from its present state of imperfection".[167] It was not a deficiency of facts but the entanglement of these facts with the theory of vital properties that was retarding the science of physiology; for, as Magendie wrote, "it is often necessary to swallow a multitude of more or less absurd explanations and sometimes of supposed or ill-observed facts in order to reach any sure and significant data in the works on physiology".[168]

How could this explanatory framework of vital properties appear to the older physiologists to be firmly based and soundly built—indeed to be the very construction of nature itself; while to Magendie it seemed only to be an "unsteady scaffolding" that his new interpretation of life "would permit . . . to collapse of its own weight"? In order to answer this question we must examine the epistemological bases of both the system of vital properties and the system of physiological explanation proposed by Magendie to replace it.

THE EPISTEMOLOGY OF VITAL PROPERTIES. The theory of vital properties originated with the concept of "irritability," which was introduced into physiology by the English physician Francis Glisson (1597–1677). The term "irritability" was first used, in an offhand fashion, in Glisson's *Anatomia hepatis* of 1654. But in his *Tractatus de ventriculo et intestinis* of 1677, he employed the term in a systematic way to refer to a general property inherent in all living matter.[169] This generalization of the Galenic concept of irritation represented a theoretical break with the past; it required, as Temkin noted, a "philosophical reorientation" on Glisson's part.[170] "No one," wrote Haller in his *Bibliotheca anatomica,* "thought correctly about irritability before Glisson."[171]

The theory of vital properties was an unchallenged feature of physiology from its introduction by Glisson until the attack mounted against it in the first decade of the nineteenth century. It underlay the great physiological controversies for more than a hundred years and defined the theoretical boundaries within which they were disputed. Mechanists, vitalists, and animists offered competing explanations of the vital properties;[172] and when Haller and the Montpellier physicians debated methodology, the argument centered on how best to study these properties.[173]

The vital properties, then, were central to the theoretical problematic of physiology throughout the period known as the classical age—extending from about 1660 to about 1800–10. This period was characterized by a distinctive epistemology, and in the present section of our study we shall attempt to show the relationship of this epistemology to the theoretical problematic of vital properties and its methodological correlate, the research problematic of observation.

Within the epistemology of the classical period knowledge appeared as *order*—an atemporal, tabular order established by the application of the universal method of analysis. We have already seen, at the beginning of part two of this study, that Magendie referred to his own physiology as "analytical"; however, the term analysis had a special meaning for the classical epistemology that it lost at the beginning of the nineteenth century and that was foreign to Magendie's way of thought.

Analysis, for the empirical, nonmathematical sciences of the classical age, meant the discrimination of sensible differences. The phenomena to be studied would first be considered as a whole and the major components distinguished. These components, in turn, would be divided into their constituent parts, with the process continuing until the "elements" of the phenomena—the least differences perceptible—had been reached. Finally, these elementary components would be reassembled in their proper order, giving a complete understanding of the complex phenomena in terms of the nature and interrelation of their constituents. The efficacy of this type of analysis was predicated upon the tacit presupposition that the hidden system of nature was faithfully represented to the senses by the observable properties of things, and that these properties could be interpreted as a system of signs.[174] Hence the classical epistemology authorized the research problematic of observation by guaranteeing that the unprejudiced and skillful analysis of the phenomena by means of observation would yield knowledge of the true order of nature.

For physiology, such an analysis took the form of dividing the observable bodily processes into a small number of classes exhibiting distinctive common features or properties. These classes were then subdivided until their "elements"—either one or several observational properties—were reached. Such functional elements, named "vital properties" to indicate that they specifically characterized living beings, were finally correlated in various ways with the anatomical elements that the analysis of the dissection table had revealed.

The number and relative importance of the different vital properties was a matter of intense controversy throughout the classical period. For Glisson and others there was only one such property, irritability; while Haller and his adherents argued that sensibility was a separate and equally important vital property. But in France, especially during the last half of the eighteenth century, when the analysis of sensations begun by John Locke (1632–1704) reached an extreme form in the philosophy later called "sensualism," it was sensibility that became the dominant vital property.

While the *philosophe* Étienne Bonnot, abbé de Condillac (1715–80) argued in his *Essai sur l'origine des connoissances humaines* (1746) and *Traité des sensations* (1754) that all knowledge—indeed all the human mental faculties themselves—arose from sensations variously transformed,[175] Bordeu and his colleagues were elaborating a theory in which all physiological processes were regarded as arising from sensibility. After explaining glandular secretion on this basis, for example, Bordeu concluded: "Secretion is thus reduced to a kind of *sensation.*"[176] And while few other French physiologists of the period went as far as Bordeu or Fouquet in making sensibility the *unique* principle of life—the source of both sensation and motion[177]—most of them nevertheless agreed that the motion of any part presupposed the existence of some form of sensibility within that part. As Barthez wrote: "The influence of the sensitive forces seems to me to be the immediate cause of the action of the motive forces of the organs.[178] Hence the necessity for the existence of the vital property that Bichat called "organic sensibility."

The same epistemology, then, which authorized the progressive analysis of the living body into anatomical elements—organs, tissues, molecules—also produced an explanation of the processes of these elements that transferred to the physiological level the same priority that sensation enjoyed at the psychological level. The resulting "correspondence" of the two levels was celebrated at the end of the century by the physician and *idéologue* Pierre-Jean-Georges Cabanis (1757–1808) in his *Rapports du physique et du moral de l'homme* as follows:

> Surely we have no need of proving once again that physical sensibility is the source of all the ideas and all the habits which constitute the moral existence of man: Locke, Bonnet, Condillac and Helvétius have demonstrated this truth to the fullest degree. Among those who are instructed and who make any use at all of their reason, there is no one who can raise the slightest doubt in this regard. On the other hand, the physiologists have proven that all the vital movements are the product of impressions received by the sensible parts: and these two fundamental results, brought together in a reflective examination, form but one and the same truth.[179]

Such correspondences did not appear to eighteenth-century physiologists as products of an unfounded anthropomorphic assumption. To them the theory of the vital properties, however they interpreted it and whichever property they gave prominence to, was as soundly based as the Newtonian theory of gravitation, and they did not hesitate to draw this comparison explicitly.[180] Indeed the vital properties functioned within all their systems as *forces* and were regarded by them as physiological equivalents of the force of affinity in chemistry and the force of attraction in astronomy. Dumas, for example, after listing his four vital forces (sensitive force, contractile or motive force, assimilative force, and force of vital resistance) wrote: "These principles of action in living beings correspond to the four forces of *impulsion, attraction, affinity,* and *inertia* which aid in classifying the phenomena of non-living nature.''[181] And Cabanis even suggested that the gravitational force itself might be nothing else but a cosmic manifestation of sensibility.[182] Similarly, Bichat, while not equating the physical and vital properties in the manner suggested by Cabanis, nevertheless accorded them the same ontological status: "To create the universe," he stated, "God endowed matter with gravity, elasticity, affinity, etc., and furthermore one portion received as its share sensibility and contractility.''[183]

Magendie later objected to the claims of his predecessors that explanation by means of the vital properties raised physiology to the same level that Newton's work had raised the physical sciences. Newton, he pointed out, had not discovered the existence of attraction, which was already known, but rather the mathematical law according to which attraction operates in the universe. Thus, to Magendie's mind, physiology was still awaiting its Newton.[184]

But this objection would have carried no weight with the eighteenth-century physiologists, since the classical epistemology recognized the order established in the sphere of the qualitative, by the analysis of least sensible differences, as having the same scientific status as the order established by measurement and calculation in the sphere of the quantitative. Both were considered applications of the general science of order, the fir employing linguistic signs and the second numerical or algebraic symbols.[185] Quasimathematical rigor was attainable in physiology if the vital properties themselves were made more determinate by distinguishing their modifications in the different parts of the body. Thus Bichat's care to distinguish organic contractility from animal contractility, for example, and then to divide the former of these two modes into its sensible and insensible varieties, was an attempt to assure the precision of mathematics in the study of what, for him, were essentially nonquantifiable phenomena.[186]

The classical epistemology, then, was the underlying foundation of the theory of vital properties, without which that theory was truly nothing but an "unsteady scaffolding." But at the end of the eighteenth century the epistemology of the analysis of sensations was replaced by another one, of a wholly different configuration, which brought with it an organic conception of life incompatible with the previous interpretation of living phenomena. And it was this new conception of life that underlay all Magendie's criticisms of the older physiologists and all his own physiological proposals, as we shall see in the following two sections.

THE EPISTEMOLOGY OF ORGANIC FUNCTIONS. For the new epistemology that arose at the beginning of the nineteenth century, empirical knowledge was constituted in a way entirely different from that which was established by the classical epistemology. Rather then taking the form of an analytic order established by the isolation of sensible elements, empirical knowledge now began to appear as a system of internal relations between organized units that were not simply reducible to their component parts and that functioned together as a totality. Concomitant with this epistemological reorganization stressing internal relations, there arose a new conception of life and of the proper manner of studying it, for which the most prominent spokesman was the zoologist Georges Cuvier (1769–1832).[187] And as we shall see, this same conception was shared by Magendie.

It may at first seem paradoxical to link Cuvier in this way with Magendie "the inflexible experimenter,"[188] in view of the former's reputation as an opponent of vivisection. Indeed, Joseph Schiller has asserted that such a connection "defies the ABCs of physiology and of its history."[189] It is important to note, however, that Cuvier's early opposition to vivisection was limited only to "certain experiments upon living bodies"[190] in which the experimenter first removed or destroyed some vital organ from an animal and they attempted to deduce, from the phenomena of the animal's death, the role which the affected organ played in the normal state. Living bodies, he believed, "cannot be dismantled without being destroyed; we cannot know what would result from the absence of one or several of their [organs] and consequently we cannot know what part each of these [organs] plays in the total effect."[191] Thus Cuvier recommended the study of comparative anatomy as an alternative to such types of vivisectional experimentation; and he was seconded on this point by the experimental physiologist J.-J.-C. Legallois (1770–1840).[192] But when Magendie, Legallois, and Cuvier's own protégé Pierre Flourens (1794–1867) subsequently developed techniques for vivisectional experimentation, upon the neuromuscular system in particular, which depended for their success not upon the death of the animal but rather upon its survival for as long as possible, then Cuvier actively encouraged these researches and furthered the careers of those experimenters who carried out such techniques.[193]

The new conception of life, which both Cuvier and Magendie shared, presented the living creature as an organized whole, a functionally integrated system rather than an assemblage of juxtaposed organs.[194] Thus a central feature of this view of life was the elevation of functions to a status of priority over anatomical structure. Whereas the older interpretation of life had assumed a strict one-to-one correspondence between structure and function— each part having its special use and, conversely, each function having its special organ[195]—at the beginning of the nineteenth century "function" became understood as a general result to be obtained by a variety of possible anatomical means. There are very few structural features, Cuvier pointed out, which are common to all organs of a given kind throughout the animal kingdom. Often, he continued, these organs resemble each other only in the effect they produce. This must be especially striking in regard to respiration, which operates in the different classes [of animals] by means of organs so varied that their structures offer no points in common. These differences between organs of the same kind are precisely the object of comparative anatomy. . . . We are therefore going to take each one of the functions which we have just discussed and examine . . . the particular means by which it is effected in different animals.[196]

For Cuvier this functional conception of life provided the key to a new system of classification (and a new science of paleontology) based upon comparative anatomy; for it was now "toward the functions themselves rather than toward the organs" that the naturalist's attention must be directed in the search for valid taxonomic characters.[197] And it was this same conception of life, with its focus on functions rather than organs, which furnished Magendie with a new guiding principle for the study of physiology.

Magendie defined the "true function" in his theoretical paper of 1809 as "the common end of the actions of a certain number of organs."[198] It was not this definition that was new, however, since Bichat had propounded it in nearly the same terms in his lectures of the year X (1801–02) when he told his students that "one organ alone does not carry out a function; a function is thus the result of the labor of several organs. In the animal economy there is a great number of organs which appertain to several apparatuses."[199] And in his *Anatomie descriptive* the same concept of function was implied when he defined an "apparatus" as "an assemblage of several organs contributing to one function," and added shortly afterward that "nature often causes the same [organs] to serve entirely different functions."[200] In the past, wrote Bichat in the same work, the organs of animals had been described according to the region of the body in which they were located, but this procedure constituted only a topographical anatomy for use by surgeons and artists. The advance of physiology, however, made it necessary to group the organs into apparatuses and describe them according to the functions to which they contributed. "Citizens Cuvier and Dumeril," he concluded, "have also chosen the functions as the character by which to classify the organs of animals. I shall follow the same procedure; it is the only one which can be adopted in our present state of knowledge."[201]

It was not Magendie, then, but Bichat who broke with the traditional concept of a function as the unique action of a single organ.[202] And Magendie indicated that he recognized the equivalence of his concept of function with Bichat's when he adopted the latter's term "apparatus" in his *Précis élémentaire* as, for example, when he spoke of giving a "summary anatomical description of the organs which contribute to the function, or of the apparatus."[203]

This new concept of function that Bichat, perhaps borrowing from the comparative anatomy of Féliz Vicq-d'Azyr (1748–94),[204] introduced into physiology was wholly integrated into his theoretical problematic of vital properties. Under the analytic interpretation of life, which this problematic presupposed, the vital phenomena manifested by the organism as a whole were regarded purely as the sum of the phenomena of the more or less autonomous elementary parts of the living body. For Bordeu, these anatomical elements were the organs, each of which he considered to have a life of its own. "Thus," he wrote,

the least part may be regarded as forming, so to speak, a separate body [*corps à part*]. . . . In order to appreciate properly the particular action of each part, let us compare the living body to a swarm of bees which gathers into little clusters and which hangs from a tree like a bunch of grapes. The saying of a celebrated Ancient, that one of the viscera of the lower abdomen was an animal within an animal, has met with approval: each part is, so to speak, undoubtedly not an animal but rather a kind of separate machine which contributes in its fashion *to the general life* of the body.[205]

But Bichat pushed Bordeu's anatomical analysis farther and, in his *Anatomie générale,* isolated twenty-one simple tissues—each having a life of its own—which, by their various combinations comprised the different organs.[206] And since, for Bichat, an organ was a composite of several different tissues, each of which enjoyed a variety of vital properties in differing degrees, he had no trouble in conceiving of the activities of the organs as contributing to several different functions. Nevertheless, he strictly adhered to the analytic interpretation of life, insisting that the study of the simple tissue systems (general anatomy) was an "essential introduction" to the study of the organs (descriptive anatomy) and that this latter undertaking was a necessary "first step in the study of the functions" to which these organs contributed (physiology).[207]

For Magendie, however, it was not the properties and activities of the anatomical elements, whether organs or tissues, which ought to occupy the focal point of physiology, but rather the functions themselves. Thus his order of research was precisely the opposite of Bichat's. "The mode of studying a particular function," he wrote,

is not a matter of indifference. The following is that which we adopt.
1. The general idea of the function.
2. The circumstances which put the organs into action, and which we shall denominate, *excitants of the function.*
3. The summary anatomical description of the organs which contribute to the function, or of the apparatus.
4. The study of the action of each organ in particular [as it relates to the function].
5. General recapitulation, showing the utility of the function.
6. The relation of the function with those previously examined.

7. The modifications of the functions according to age, sex, temperament, climate, seasons and habit.[208]

As Bichat had understood it, the "unit" of physiology was still the anatomical element, whose various observable properties combined with those of other elements to produce different functions in the way that various integers combined to produce different sums. But Magendie's "unit" was the function, conceived of as the specific result effected by a particular organic structure—a totality of organs and processes considered only insofar as they produced the function in question. The function, on this understanding, was an abstract relationship, a "general idea," in which the observable properties of anatomical parts played no part. The function could not be approached by a process of anatomical deduction; the contribution of each participating organ had to be experimentally determined. Hence Magendie's reliance upon a research problematic of experimentation.[209]

Magendie's research memoirs were typically organized so as to take one of the functions as a starting point and to trace it back experimentally to the organs contributing to it[210] (i.e., steps 1–4 in Magendie's list; steps 5–7 being reserved for the more comprehensive exposition of the textbook). Thus in his memoir on absorption, as we have seen, he sought to demonstrate that the function of absorption in mammals was carried out not only by the lymphatic system but also by the venous system.[211] The experimental technique he employed in this research, as we have also seen, was precisely that used by Bichat in his studies on respiration, but the conception of the relationship between a vital function and its anatomical substrate was entirely new. And it was this new conception that liberated physiology from anatomy.[212]

Also new was the conception of physiological analogies, which similarly were no longer based upon observable properties of bodily parts, but upon functional relations. Indeed, it was this very manner of regarding analogies that made it possible for Magendie to employ the same experiments that Bichat had carried out on respiration and asphyxiation in his own study of absorption; for the absorption of nutriments or injected substances and the entry of inhaled gases into the bloodstream were analogous processes to Magendie: "aliments, drinks, medicines, and the air itself do not become useful to us until they have been absorbed."[213] For Bichat, on the other hand, the only connection between absorption and respiration was at the level of the vital properties that enabled the organs involved to carry out these functions properly. "The absorption of the lacteal vessels," wrote Bichat,

which in their ordinary state [of sensibility] introduce into the blood only nutritive substances, can thus often be an open portal to a mass of morbific principles [when their sensibility is altered]. Similarly the vessels in the lungs, which take from the air substances appropriate for coloring the blood, often take principles which are fatal to the functions, according to the diverse alterations which the sensibility of these vessels can experience.[214]

It was the analogy of the vital properties that interested Bichat; the analogy of respiration and absorption as general processes was invisible to him.

NUTRITION AND ACTION. With the new primacy of functions over anatomical elements came a series of changes in the interpretation of life—changes which can be observed in parallel forms in the systems of Cuvier and Magendie. Within the theoretical problematic of function the terms of the older problematic of vital properties took on new meanings. "Sensibility" and "contractility," for example, were no longer understood as causal entities; for Cuvier and Magendie these two terms, where applicable at all, simply designated effects—that is, the functions "sensation" and "contraction."[215] Related to this development was the disappearance of the priority that the epistemology of analysis had conferred upon sensations. Thus Cuvier denounced "the sort of contradiction and metaphysical obscurity that must necessarily be entailed by a pretended local sensibility without perception which is admitted in particular organs by all [Montpellier] physicians and defended even today [1808] by some of them."[216] And Magendie likewise dismissed "local" or "organic" sensibility as a gratuitous and empty hypothesis.

It was no longer sensation but nutrition that occupied the status of priority among the physiological processes in the systems of Cuvier and Magendie. Cuvier described life as "a continuous whirlpool whose direction, complicated though it is, remains constant, as does the type of molecules which are caught up in it, although not the individual molecules themselves,"[217] and he went on to note that "The first point which strikes us in the study of life is that force which organized bodies have for attracting into their whirlpools foreign substances, for retaining them there a while after assimilating them, and finally for distributing to all their parts these substances which have become their own, according to the functions which must be exercised in each."[218] Similarly, Magendie set out as his first point "that living bodies take from the substances in the midst [*milieu*] of which they live, and carry to their interiors, a certain quantity of matter which generally bears the name of *nutritive matter* or *aliment*."[219]

Finally, the elimination of sensibility and contractility as causal concepts necessitated a new explanation of the variety of particular processes carried out by the bodily organs. Cuvier suggested an explanation based upon the production and consumption of an imponderable fluid that he called the "nervous agent";[220] but Magendie seemed to reject this approach when he attacked "the truly ridiculous supposition of a nervous fluid circulating through the nerves—a supposition which inadvertently recalls the infancy of physiology.''[221] Nevertheless, Magendie was faced with the same problem as Cuvier even though he proposed a different answer—indeed the answer he proposed shows him to have been, in a sense, *plus royaliste que le roi;* for where Cuvier adapted a concept from contemporary chemistry, Magendie adapted one from Cuvier's comparative anatomy.

Magendie's solution to the problem was to assert that the activity of an organ is the consequence of "the nature, the disposition and the mode of union of the living molecules—in a word, their organization.''[222] Such an explanation was, of course, simply the transference to the molecules, in their relation to the activity of the organ, of a principle which Cuvier applied to the organs, in their relation to the activity of the organism as a whole. And Magendie explicitly drew this comparison:

> It is, in my opinion, extremely probable that if our means of investigating anatomical structures are developed in the future to a high degree of perfection, we will be able to account for the nuances of life as well as we now account for its great differences. With what marvelous facility do the zoologists succeed in determining, in a rigorous manner, all the phenomena of the life of an animal, simply by considering one of its organs—a tarsal bone, for example! I consider this part of zoology to be one of the most remarkable and most satisfying things which has ever been accomplished.[223]

Magendie's explanation of the actions of the various organs was an adaptation of Cuvier's principle of the "correlation of parts." This principle held that

> all the organs of a given animal form a unique system in which all the parts act, react, and are connected with one another; and there cannot be any modification in one of those parts without bringing about analogous modifications in all the others.
> It is upon this principle that the method is founded which Mr. Cuvier has conceived for recognizing an animal by a single bone, by a single facet of a bone.[224]

Cuvier derived his principle of the correlation of parts from his consideration of what he called the "conditions of existence" of each animal species. Only certain combinations of organs were physiologically compatible with one another, therefore the presence of a certain type of bone structure implied a certain type of digestive system, a certain method of locomotion, and so on. Hence the correlation of parts was a reflection of the internal conditions of existence of each species.

There were also external conditions of existence to be considered, however. These, for Cuvier, were given by the relationship between the animal and the physical *milieu* surrounding it, from which it continually assimilated molecules by alimentation, by absorption through its skin, and by respiration.[225] Here, then, we have the key to the priority that nutrition assumed in Magendie's physiological system, for Magendie once again transferred to the molecules of the living body, in their relationship to the organs, a principle which Cuvier applied to the organs in their relationship to the animal as a whole.

Thus Magendie's proposed interpretation of life was an adaptation to physiology of the Cuverian notion of the conditions of existence; it laid down the same requirements at the physiological level that Cuvier's system posited for the existence of a species. For Cuvier these requirements were the internal coordination of the organs so as to make possible the harmonious exercise of all the necessary functions of life, and also the suitability of those organs (considered as a whole system) in relation to their environment (considered as a source of materials for nutrition and respiration). For Magendie these same requirements demanded the internal coordination (organization) of the molecules of each organ so as to allow that organ to perform its appropriate action, and also the ability of those molecules (considered as a whole organ) to nourish themselves in proportion to their degree of activity. "Vital action," Magendie wrote in his *Précis,* "depends evidently upon nutrition, and nutrition again is influenced by vital action. Thus an organ which ceases to be nourished, loses at the same time the faculty of acting; thus organs whose action is the most frequently repeated, have a more active nutrition: on the contrary, those which act less, have evidently a sluggish nutritive movement."[226]

Magendie's application of the Cuvierian principle of the conditions of existence to the organs and their constituent molecules had momentous consequences for the development of physiology in the nineteenth century, only one of which we shall mention here by way of illustration. Just as an animal species that can no longer get its requisite food must become extinct, so too "an organ which ceases to be nourished, loses at the same time the faculty of acting." From the first of these considerations Cuvier concluded that the *milieu* of a species must remain constant for the species to survive in it (otherwise the species must either perish or emigrate). The second of these considerations implied (although Magendie did not himself make the inference) that the living molecules of the body also required a constant *milieu* for their maintenance; it thus provided a necessary precondition for Claude Bernard's later elaboration of the concept of the *milieu intérieur.*[227]

CONCLUSION. We have shown that all Magendie's criticisms of the older explanatory system of vital properties, and all his own proposals for physiological explanation, were based upon a new conception of life that appeared at the beginning of the nineteenth century. From the point of view of this new conception, which represented a theoretical break with the classical interpretation of life, physiology was "still in its infancy" in 1816 because it was essentially starting anew—it was, according to Magendie, in the condition of physics at the time of Galileo and Bacon rather than at the time of

Newton.[228] Or, if we wish to use chemistry as a basis of comparison instead of physics, we may say that Magendie's *Précis élémentaire de physiologie* was the equivalent of Lavoisier's *Traité élémentaire de chimie* (1789) both in self-conscious design and in objective relationship to its science.[229] The historical significance of Magendie's *Précis,* then, lay not just in its consistent application of the experimental method, as Claude Bernard thought,[230] but more importantly in its status as the first textbook embodying the new theoretical problematic of physiology.

A certain amount of factual data could be retained from the physiology of vital properties, but these facts had to be (1) confirmed, chiefly by new experiments,[231] (2) integrated into the functional conception of life, and (3) augmented by a vast amount of new experimental research carried out within the problematic of function, before any comprehensive science of physiology would be possible. Physiology, once liberated from anatomical deduction by the problematic of function, required an experimental method, because the functions to be studied were no longer simply deducible from the observable properties of anatomical parts, but were processes—variously effected in various classes of animals—that depended upon a complex set of internal relations. Magendie's *extreme* positivism in his later career was probably motivated, as Georges Canguilhem has suggested,[232] by political considerations; but the experimental method in physiology arose at the beginning of the nineteenth century from something far more integral to the science itself than Magendie's personality.

As Canguilhem himself has put it, "The problem [of experimentation] in biology . . . is not one of utilizing experimental concepts, but one of experimentally constituting concepts which are authentically biological."[233] We have seen that Bichat applied experimental concepts in his investigation of living organisms, but this investigation itself depended upon the theoretical problematic of vital properties, utilizing concepts borrowed partly from Newtonian physics (e.g., forces, "atomic" analysis) and partly from Lockean psychology (e.g., sensibility), with the anthropomorphic element derived from the latter particularly evident. Within the new theoretical problematic of the nineteenth century, however, the idea of organic function was a purely biological concept, dependent neither upon physics nor psychology. And it was the constitution of this concept—theoretically by Cuvier and experimentally by Magendie—that definitely established the experimental method in physiology, beginning the revolution that Claude Bernard was to complete.[234]

The simplistic portrayal of Magendie's achievement in experimental physiology as a personal triumph over Bichat's vitalism, which we owe to Claude Bernard[235] and to subsequent historians who have seen things through his eyes, can thus no longer be accepted. Rather than thinking in terms of personalities and their individual contributions, we must approach the birth of a new science of physiology at the beginning of the nineteenth century as a regional effect within a more general reorganization of certain non-mathematized forms of knowledge that was occurring at that time in western culture.[236] Taking this approach, as we have done, cannot in itself produce a fully adequate account of the appearance of a new physiology, however; for the larger transformation of knowledge in which we have attempted to situate this appearance was undoubtedly determined, in the last instance, by a system of relations lying outside the domain of knowledge entirely. A complete and satisfactory account of the birth of a new physiology, or of any new science, must await a theory explaining the successive alterations that the fabric of knowledge itself has undergone. The elaboration of such a theory, which thus far exists only in rudimentary form,[237] remains the principal task of intellectual history.

Acknowledgments

This study owes its origin to questions raised by William Coleman in his seminar on the history of biology at the Johns Hopkins University in 1968. Research was carried out in 1972–73 at the Johns Hopkins Institute of the History of Medicine under the supervision of Lloyd Stevenson, director of the Institute, and was supported by a generous postdoctoral fellowship from the Josiah Macy, Jr., Foundation.

At various stages in its development this work was read and commented on by the following persons, whose assistance is gratefully acknowledged: Dr. Stevenson and Dr. Coleman at Johns Hopkins; Dr. David Oldroyd and Dr. Guy Freeland, my colleagues in the School of History and Philosophy of Science at the University of New South Wales; and Dr. Camille Limoges, director of the Institut d'histoire et de sociopolitique des sciences at the Université de Montréal, who also was kind enough to check the accuracy of my translations of the texts by Bichat and Magendie included in the appendix.

A portion of the material contained in the second part of this study was previously published in the *Bulletin of the History of Medicine,* 48(1974), and is incorporated here with the permission of the editor.

Appendix

TEXTS

1. Bichat, *Discourse on the Study of Physiology,* 1798.
2. Cuvier, *On the Use of the Vital Principle in Physiology,* 1806.
3. Magendie, *Some General Ideas on the Phenomena Peculiar to Living Bodies,* 1809.

DISCOURSE ON THE STUDY OF PHYSIOLOGY
by Xavier Bichat[238]

1. Definition of physiology.

2. It is composed of the study of phenomena and the study of causes. The first is founded upon observation and the second upon reasoning; every physiological question presents these two aspects, [for] example; respiration, digestion;—first one observes and then one explains what one has observed.

3. Analogy of physiology with the physical sciences: astronomy, physics. 1st observation, 2nd explanation; this is the ordinary sequence.

4. Hence in physiological study: the history of the phenomena and the history of the theories. A phenomenon is that which meets the eye; a theory, that which explains.

5. Certainty, precision of the first part of physiology; [in contrast to the] often fanciful uncertainty of the second.

6. Division of this discourse: to examine 1st, the part of physiology [which is] founded upon observation; 2nd, the part [which is] founded upon reasoning.

FIRST PART—OBSERVATIONAL PHYSIOLOGY[239]

Observational physiology preceded rational physiology. The ancients knew only the phenomena which they observed; they followed the same procedure here as [they did] in medicine—recall *Hippocratic medicine;*[240]—a long time was required for amassing facts before rational physiology was attained. Thus their physiological knowledge was certain, [it contained] nothing hypothetical, but the science was advanced very little. The moderns, while adding theories, have not neglected observation; they have collected new facts, established new hypotheses. The question here is to examine the sources from which the facts must be drawn; now there are three means: 1st, observation of healthy men [and animals]; 2nd, experiments upon living animals; 3rd, observations upon diseased [men and] animals.

1. OBSERVATION OF HEALTHY [MEN AND] ANIMALS

This is the first method of observation which offers itself; it is the simplest and the most natural. It is this method which reveals to us two great classes of functions: the one external and the other internal. It is this method which reveals to us that the exterior life is composed: 1st, of the action of the senses, of sensations; 2nd, of perception by the brain; 3rd, of the will and the judgment; 4th, of locomotion.

It is this method which reveals to us a double movement in the interior life—[one] of composition by means of the nutrients and [one] of decomposition by means of the excrements, perspiration, insensible transpiration, etc.

But in order for this observation of the healthy animal to be effective it must be conjoined with anatomical knowledge. Without this science we would only have vague notions of the exterior and interior life; we would have no data at all about the agents of these functions or even about their division. Without anatomy we would not know the diverse functions which compose the interior life: *the internal secretion, exhalation and absorption* would be unknown.

Thus anatomy must everywhere join with the observation of the phenomena of the healthy animal.

It is the lack of this union between anatomy and the observation of phenomena to which must be attributed the small scope of the ancients' knowledge in physiology, even though they observed very well—although the physicians of Montpellier regarded the science [of physiology] in a philosophical manner, they would have caused it to make more progress if they had known more anatomy—Haller caused it to make such great progress only because of this.

Man must not be studied in an isolated manner, but the functions must be observed in the different species of animals; it is necessary to observe;

Respiration in animals with $\left\{\begin{array}{l}\text{trachea,}\\ \text{gills,}\\ \text{lungs.}\end{array}\right.$

Circulation in animals with $\left\{\begin{array}{l}\text{general circulation.}\\ \text{capillary circulation, only [class] known: the}\\ \quad\text{zoophytes;}\\ \text{among animals with general circulation,}\\ \quad\text{it is necessary to see}\\ \quad\text{those whose hearts have}\end{array}\right.$ $\left\{\begin{array}{l}\text{one ventricle;}\\ \text{two ventricles, etc.}\end{array}\right.$

In [the case of] sensibility $\left\{\begin{array}{l}\text{animals with a brain;}\\ \text{animals without a brain.}\end{array}\right.$

Etc.[241]

2. EXPERIMENTS ON LIVING ANIMALS

The ancients performed no experiments upon living animals, or at least very few; they dissected dogs and calves, as one sees in Galen, Erasistratus and Herophilus, but the goal of this dissection was anatomy much more than physiology. Since the discovery of the circulation, of the [. . .][242] of respiration some individuals have singularly multiplied these experiments. Thereupon, in the school of Montpellier, others protested against them, so that the first group believe that physiology can only advance by means of experiments while the others believe that they are fruitless.[243] From what does this difference of opinion arise? The cause of it is that the subject has been regarded in too general a manner; in some cases experiments are advantageous, and in others they are very uncertain, etc.

I. *The Uncertainty of Experiments*.—This uncertainty is noted above all when the experiments have the vital forces as their object. The animal, agitated and fearful, goes into spasms or convulsions; its irritability and sensibility are no longer the same, everything in the [animal] economy which relates to the vital forces undergoes a change. So true [is] this that there are some contradictory experiments by Haller in the case of the sensibility of the dura mater.[244] Besides, one of the remarkable laws of this property is that it can be transported from one place to another; now in these transportations of sensibility one cannot very well grasp its character. One must, therefore, exercise great restraint in making pronouncements about the vital forces based upon experiments.

[II.] *The Certainty of Experiments*.—But there is a multitude of other circumstances in which experiments give us very certain notions.

Examples:

1. Digestion—experiments of Spallanzani.[245]—My experiments upon the gall-bladder;[246]

2. Respiration, various asphyxias; etc.[247]

3. Absorption, causing fluids to be absorbed;[248]

4. Influence of the secretions upon one another;[249]

5. Nutrition of the bones. Experiment of [. . .],[250] etc.

In all of these cases the experiments are certain; invariable results are drawn from them; but they demand extreme precision. It is difficult to set out general rules, but here are a few nonetheless:

1. Object of comparison. [For example] one must always compare the state of a healthy animal with that of the animal upon which one experiments.

[1.] Falsity of the experiments of Lieutaud upon the spleen.[251]

2. Emphysema by oxygen and by pure air for the coloring of the blood.[252]

2. Do not attribute to one cause what is due to a foreign cause. Example: what happened to me in making a guinea-pig emphysematic by oxygen—sudden death. Sometimes carbonic acid [gas] kills, although it is nevertheless not poisonous.[253]

3. Repeat several experiments with the same object: only from a number [of experiments] can truth result, because the animal might be in circumstances which prevent [the success of] the experiment in one case; example: extirpation of the spleen. I have tried this experiment three times this year without success. 1st Inflammation of the lower abdomen; 2nd pinching of the intestine; 3rd the spleen eaten away.

4. Consider the state of the animal, etc.

3. OBSERVATION OF DISEASES

The ancients observed [diseases] very well; the moderns have neglected this means [of study] somewhat. Nevertheless it is essential. It is necessary to examine the advantages which physiology draws from medicine. These advantages are not at all as substantial as they seem at first. In order to distinguish these advantages adequately it is necessary to divide diseases into *organic* and *general* diseases.

[*Organic Diseases.*]—The majority of the organic diseases cast much light upon physiology (I understand by organic disease anything that disturbs the organization).

Example: cataracts, pressure on the brain, concussions, scirrhus of the pylorus, stones in the gall-bladder, aneurism of the heart, etc., pressure of a tumor on the thoracic duct, etc.

In all these cases pathology furnishes physiology[254] with essential data; the facts must be collected with precision.

General Diseases.—These diseases furnish fewer physiological data than the others. Example: fever has not advanced our knowledge of the circulation at all. Above all those diseases which attack the vital forces do little to illuminate the theory of those forces. There is no relation between the sensibility which has been observed in experiments and the nervous or vaporous affections. Consider the innumerable phenomena of diseases. It is impossible to relate them to the known laws of sensibility—not only to relate them to the known laws but even to found new laws upon these phenomena; because they do not resemble each other, they are all different and are diversely modified in diverse parts and in diverse affections. Note the nervous affections of women, the phenomena of the malignant fever, the putrid fever, etc.

Often the irritation occurs at one point and the contraction at another. Whence the term sympathy, a word which serves to veil our ignorance of the connection which links these phenomena.[255] Why does the diaphragm contract when the nose is irritated? Because, it is said, there is a sympathy between them. But what is this sympathy? To what is it due? In the final analysis we have little data on diseases to compare with the phenomena of the healthy state.

SECOND PART—RATIONAL PHYSIOLOGY. THEORIES

In the first part I showed the foundations upon which physiology must be based and from which the history of the phenomena, or observational physiology, must be drawn. But the phenomena must be coordinated, their totality must be sought out. The mind of man, naturally curious, seeks causes; thus[256] rational physiology soon came into being. One sought to explain what one had observed; whence theories, hypotheses and explanations were born.

1. Explanation concerns an isolated phenomenon.

2. Hypothesis concerns a greater number of phenomena and assumes a plan, but the hypothesis is not founded upon anything certain; it is a system, it imagines causes.

[3.] Theory is founded upon facts, upon experiments; it is a statement, a result of a mass of facts; and in this it differs from a hypothesis. For example, in the system [of] digestion: 1st, suction of fluids is an explanation; 2nd, fermentation of acids is a hypothesis; 3rd, dissolution is a theory—for example Spallanzani [. . .][257]—or the theories of [. . .].[257]

General rule: explanations ought to be accommodated to general theories, to enter into them. Hypotheses must be banished; there must only be theories which encompass a great [number][258] of facts.

GENERAL RULE FOR THEORIES

1. A theory must never reach beyond secondary causes. Any ultima ratio is forbidden to us; the veil must not[259] be raised. Example: the difference between the present and the ancient modes of philosophizing about generation.

2. It must be in conformity with the vital laws, it must be in accord with the other functions. General principle of the animal economy: nature is frugal in means, prodigal in results.[260] For example, when we see all the mucous[261] membranes exhaling and absorbing [fluids], if someone wants to propose to us a theory for a single one of these membranes in which the separation of the fluid occurs differently [than in the other mucous membranes, then this theory is suspect]; for example, those who claim that the humor of the chest is formed by great [. . .].[262]—The analogy with perspiration testifies in favor of [its formation by] the pulmonary exhalation; Lavoisier wants to establish another theory, [but] it has against it the general course of nature.[263]—I see the mucous juices everywhere given off outwards; if, in a theory of digestion someone makes them return inwards, this theory is suspect, etc.

3. Whence follows a very simple consequence, which is that every theory must be founded upon a great number of facts. Thus every theory of absorption, or of the secretions, etc., ought to have been the fruit of the observation of a great number of [absorptive or] secretory organs. Hence the advantage of comparative anatomy.[264] Another comparative anatomy [studies the same organ] at different ages.

4. The consequences must agree with the principles. Discuss here the correct manner of reasoning.

THE RELATIONSHIP OF PHYSIOLOGY WITH THE [OTHER] SCIENCES

We have just revealed the most advantageous manner of reasoning correctly and of establishing solid theories; but without the assistance of the accessory sciences we often cannot establish these theories upon facts and reasonings. Since nature governs living bodies by analogous laws, all the sciences which have living bodies as their object must aid the physiologist. Since nature applies the physical laws to living bodies it is necessary to know these laws. It is thus essential to give you a precise and exact idea of the relationship of physiology with all the [other] sciences.

Note in passing how all the sciences are linked together, etc.

All the sciences are divided into the moral and the physical sciences.

Moral sciences.—At first glance it seems that physiology, which is entirely occupied with matter, cannot be connected with the intellectual sciences. However I observe that there is as much of a relationship with them as there is with the physical sciences, and even more. Not all branches of physiology are equally connected with [the intellectual sciences]. Life must be divided into two: *exterior life* and *interior life*. It is only the order of the exterior life—namely sensation and perception—which is connected with metaphysics.

Speak here of Cabanis.[265]

Since Locke and Condillac found the source of our ideas in the senses,[266] it has become essential to understand these senses; it is necessary, in the theory of the brain, to understand the intimate senses: imagination, memory—all these questions are shared equally by the metaphysician and the physiologist. Advantages of the *physiologist-metaphysician:* he not only understands the senses, but he also knows that their faculty of receiving impressions varies and he understands the laws of sensensibility; he allies these laws with metaphysics which receives great assistance from them. Example: enfeeblement after a meal.

Moral [affections].—History of the passions, [which are] very different from the sensations. The sensations affect the senses, they have their seat in the brain; the passions affect the epigastric center.

The actor performing in the theater places his hand over his heart, etc., in order to express joy or love. In order to recollect, to reflect, he places it on his head,[267] etc. The passions are thus a general modification of the organic life. All the organs of the life of relation[268] remain unchanged; it is only the organic life [which is altered]. Insist upon this point.

Politics, religion, mores.

Physical sciences.—In the preceding lecture we examined the relations between the moral sciences and physiology; today it remains for us to examine its relations with the physical sciences. Since these sciences have successively been employed in physiology I shall examine them in a more particular manner. The physical sciences were little advanced among the ancients. The better they knew how to observe, the less they applied themselves to divining [causes]; perhaps it is to their ignorance of the physical sciences that the exactness of their observations must be attributed. For they applied themselves to observing, not being able to apply themselves to seeking out causes. In addition, another cause is that everything was new to them; everything struck them with wonderment,[269] whereas for us the observable phenomena are commonplace; there are no more discoveries to make, etc.

Whatever may be the cause of this difference between the ancients and us, the moderns soon applied the physical sciences to physiology. I shall not pause to show you the connection with the remoter sciences such as natural history, etc. I merely observe in passing that vegetable physiology presents the greatest connection with animal physiology. Vegetables are organized, they live; only they do not exist in a relationship with exterior bodies; but their circulatory and respiratory phenomena, etc., have many analogies [with the organic functions of animals]. What takes place in one group can thus illuminate what occurs in the other; indeed since life is simpler and less complicated among the vegetables, it seems, on the contrary, that it may be with them that we should begin.

RELATIONSHIP WITH PHYSICS [AND CHEMISTRY]

I pass over the sciences which have fewer relations with physiology in order to come to physics and chemistry. They form two great epochs in the history [of physiology]: the first includes the time which elapsed from Boerhaave to the middle of this century; then people began to sense the vacuousness of mechanical hypotheses and to reason according to the vital forces which had been more specially studied. Finally today, when chemistry has made new progress, it seems that people wish to clothe physiology in chemistry just as they had clothed it in physics. I am going to examine the degree to which these sciences can advance the science of man.

[A] *Relationship of physics with physiology.*—Physics was enthusiastically cultivated in the last century. After [. . .],[270] Galileo, and Gassendi had prepared its brilliant successes, Newton added the crowning touch, carrying this science to previously unknown heights. Physics was then what chemistry is for us today: it seemed to have issued suddenly from nothing. The impulsion of all these great men carried all minds over to their side, for—take note, citizens—the route which the great men follow is always [subsequently] that of the common people:

> *medicine at the time of Boerhaave;*
> *surgery at the time of the Academy;*
> *present-day chemistry.*

Thus people vied with one another to apply physics to physiology. Each one hastened to multiply the applications. (Point out here that the vital forces were entirely neglected, that everything seemed to be a mechanical machine.)

1. *Mechanics.*—Looking at the animal machine, who would not believe that mechanics must secure its most useful results in that area? Throughout the body there are levers of the first, second and third classes. These levers seem to be everywhere. There are [also] pullies. Example: the greater trochanter, the tendons sliding under the fibula, etc. At first glance it seems that everthing must be submitted to calculation, that one can calculate precisely the forces of our [anatomical] machines; for, as you know, people have succeeded in expressing [the forces of] all machines in algebraic formulas. Borelli simplified this labor; he wrote an extemely voluminous book in order to prove these forces [mathematically]; he calculated precisely all the muscular efforts.[271] These calculations are true but the principle from which they start is false because the forces of the muscles vary at each instant, so that there is not a single instant in which

there are not variations. Nothing can be calculated in that way.[272] So true is this that there were enormous differences between [different calculations of] the forces of the heart. Besides, the vital forces vary not only in the same individual, but also according to age, sex and temperament. No individual has them in exactly the same degree as the next individual. They vary in [different parts of] the same individual: bakers have stronger arms, dancers have [stronger] thigh-muscles, etc. Thus no base can be established. Thus you see that mechanics is not so great an aid [to physiology] as it is said to be; it is sufficient to know the principle levers, etc.

[2.] *Hydraulics.*—Looking at the fluids circulating in channels throughout [the body], traversing [it] in a thousand ways, who would not believe that all these parts could be submitted to the same calculation? Boerhaave believed this; his famous system of inflammation is entirely founded upon hydraulic laws.[273] Jurin, Keill, Sauvages, etc.—also attempted to determine [hydraulic laws] by the circulation.[274] When Harvey made the circulation known, every thing was mechanical application, but soon people were disabused. It is quite far from being the case that the circulation takes place as if through inert tubes which always follow the same movement; here are the essential differences:

1. Passions quickly change the circulation;

2. A point of irritation causes an afflux of blood, contrary to the laws of ordinary circulation;

3. Capillary circulation is outside the circulatory passages; it is entirely submitted to tonic forces;

4. Fevers, diseases, etc.

Thus we must not conceive, as did Harvey, that the circulation is carried out in a precise and rigorous manner, as it would be in a machine formed of arteries and veins and to which a piston could be adapted to represent the heart. There is a continual oscillation, a balance which the forces of life unceasingly modify, etc.

[3.] *Hydrostatics.*—Hydrostatics, the goal of which is the equilibrium of liquids, has a less evident influence upon the animal economy, in which the fluids are rarely motionless, except in the sanguine and lymphatic effusions, etc. Nevertheless syphons have still been applied to the study of the animal economy; for example: Petit [applied them] to [the study of] the eye[275]—absorption, the phenomena of the capillary tube. But if [hydrostatics] does have any influence it is almost nil; the force of life causes everything to vary.

[4.] *Theory of the air.*—1st, Application to respiration. Ancient theory of the air in which elasticity is destroyed by respiration: this theory is obviously false:

2nd, Application to the mechanical pressure upon the body. This pressure has a real influence in certain circumstances. Example: cupping-glasses, vapors, etc.

[5.] *Electricity.*—When this singular fluid became known it was applied to the organic economy. Everything was transformed into electricity. [There are] certain animals which give [electrical] phenomena: cats, etc.; torpedo-fish, etc. The nervous fluid was transformed into electricity, etc. What has remained of all that?—[only] that the electrical fluid is an excitant, that it stimulates the nerves, etc. The same is true of the magnetic fluid [from] that singular stone which attracts iron and always directs itself towards the north, etc. [It] had only a slight use in the economy [of life]; it was generally recognized that it was a sedative, etc.

[6.] *Acoustics, optics, voice.*—Let us admit it, there is no real application of physics to the organic economy except for acoustics and optics. This is not surprising: the eyes were made for light, the ears for sound; they are in a continual relationship with it; it was entirely necessary that nature should have accommodated the structure of the ear and the eye to the laws of the propagation of sound and light. [Speak of] the necessity of knowing these laws.

The result of the various considerations to which I have just addressed myself is that physics does not have as real an influence upon the animal economy as was first believed. That is not surprising; the bodies which are the object of physics are moved only by *gravity, elasticity, impact,* etc.

Organized bodies also obey these laws, but in addition they obey the vital laws: sensibility and motility. There is a struggle, a continual effort between the physical and the organic laws; the first laws are unceasingly modified by the second ones. Now since the vital laws can never be the object of a calculation, it is evident that mathemetics has almost no application to physiology. Insist here on the uselessness of mathematics, etc.

[B.] *Chemical Physiology.* Chemistry is applied to physiology. Today, when this science has made such great progress people seek to multiply its applications. The first one who gave an example of this was the man who had advanced chemistry the most, Lavoisier;[276] *The memoirs with Seguin,* [277] Fourcroy,[278] Jurine,[279] etc. The question is to examine what advantages physiology can draw from chemistry.

1. In the exterior functions—
    1. sense of sight
    2. [sense] of hearing }   chemistry useless
    3. [sense of] touch

    taste { chemistry has a little influence there
              { 1st degree of [. . .][280]

    odors { few data
           { _____

brain: [to sketch out][281] the structure of the brain
nerves:
muscles: fibrin; chemistry believed that it had found the principle of irritability in
          fibrin—Fourcroy[282]
[2. In the interior functions—]

DIGESTION

                              (saliva
1. analysis of the digestive fluids { bile
                              { pancreatic [fluid]
                              (gastric juice unknown
2. analysis of the gases in digestion. Jurine, *see* [. . .].[283]

CIRCULATION

                            { 1. movement of the blood
There are two things { 2. the blood itself

RESPIRATION
1. decomposition of the air
2. heat
3. contents of the blood

EXHALATION AND ABSORPTION
pulmonary exhalation

SECRETIONS

NUTRITION
It is here that chemistry has contributed the most to the progress [of physiology].

GENERATION
Analysis of the semen; but this analysis is quite frivolous. In general, all the fluids are strongly permeated with the vital forces, etc. Why is the bite of a mad animal so dangerous? Will chemistry tell us that?

ON THE USE OF THE VITAL PRINCIPLE IN PHYSIOLOGY
by Georges Cuvier[284]

M. Barthez, correspondent [of the Institute] and former professor from the same city [Montpellier], has republished his celebrated work on the *Elements of the Science of Man,*[285] which brought about in its day a fortunate revolution in physiology.

The very natural, but premature, desire to relate the phenomena of living bodies to the general laws of physics and chemistry led the physiologists of the seventeenth and the first half of the eighteenth centuries to conceive a mass of hypotheses which were as complicated as they were gratuitous and which were nevertheless still quite far from leading these physiologists to their goal.

A few good minds, disgusted by this labyrinth of contradictory suppositions, conceived of applying to living bodies the method which had so usefully been employed in physical astronomy since the time of Newton. This great man discovered that the movement of the heavenly bodies, so complicated in appearance, has as one of its principal elements the tendency of all parts of bodies toward each other according to certain laws and in a certain measure which he succeeded in determining (in a word, *universal gravitation*). And by admitting into their calculations, once and for all, this general fact which has been rigorously defined and evaluated, without seeking the cause of it, the astronomers have been able to explain effectively all the celestial phenomena in detail and with precision, and to foresee the time and place of occurrence of each one of these phenomena with even greater exactitude than could have been achieved by the most prolonged observations.

The renunciation of the search for first causes in order to devote oneself uniquely to the determination of secondary causes, or to the immediate elements of movements, has therefore been a most fortunate and fruitful idea.

Thus the physiologists were right in wishing to imitate it, and we owe the greatest recognition to M. Barthez for having engaged them in this enterprise by the example of his successes.

But today, when no one contests the utility of this method any longer, it will perhaps not be out of place to offer a few reflections on the rigor which is necessary for obtaining from it all that one ought to expect.

It would be necessary to imitate in all respects those astronomers who are not content to attribute the celestial phenomena vaguely to *attraction;* but who go on to analyze these phenomena, who show in them the part played by the attractions of each one of the different bodies involved and distinguish such phenomena from others which do not arise from these attractions; who, after having determined the measure and the laws by which these attractions act, then show by the agreement between rigorous calculation and precise observations that these laws are in fact constantly the same and do not result from any arbitrary supposition.

Now this is not at all what one does when one simply says that living bodies have a vital principle and when one attributes to this principle, without further definition, everything that one cannot otherwise explain. To believe that one has said something useful when one has said vaguely that sensibility and contractility are the effects of the vital principle, is, it seems to us, to delude others or to delude oneself with a word empty of meaning. In order to have the right to compare the use of the *vital principle* to that of *universal gravitation* it would be necessary to analyze separately each of the phenomena of life, to determine the part played in them by the ordinary laws of physics and chemistry; to compare afterwards the elements which these two sciences have not produced in each phenomenon, with those elements which similarly remain after the analysis of the other phenomena, in order to see if all these unknown elements (each one extracted, so to speak, separately from the diverse phenomena) have anything in common with each other; and finally to seek the laws which must be attributed to this common principle, if it is found that one exists, so that in combining it with the principles of the ordinary sciences it may give to all the observed phenomena of life an explanation which is satisfying to reason and which permits us to foresee in advance, with some exactitude, the phenomena which must occur in new circumstances. Only thus can physiology flatter itself with having a particular principle in the same way that astronomy has one; only thus will it be permitted by proper logic to use the *vital principle* in its reasonings and calculations as a general fact the primitive cause of which one may dispense with seeking until such time as new discoveries offer a well-founded hope of recognizing it.[286]

But one is sensible that this goal shall only be reached by perfecting the anatomy and chemistry of organized bodies,[287] by unceasingly comparing their results with the observations of these bodies both in the state of health and in the state of disease, and finally by applying this method to all classes of these bodies, whatever the complexity of their organs and the extent of their faculties.

The works on the medical and physiological sciences which are appearing daily show how necessary it was for me to recall these principles, and it would undoubtedly have been difficult for me to find a moment and place for presenting them which was more favorable than this one, in which I speak, to some extent, in the name of a body that has founded upon these principles all the important works of which I have previously given an account.

SOME GENERAL IDEAS ON THE PHENOMENA PECULIAR TO LIVING BODIES
by Dr. Magendie, Physician of the Faculty of Paris, Professor of Anatomy and Physiology, Member of the Medical Society of Emulation of Paris

The character of a certain and perfected science is that it has as its base only a small number of principles to which a great number of facts are easily connected. The physical sciences, properly so-called, generally have this character; chemistry, physics, and above all astronomy, are noteworthy examples of it. The physiological sciences, having many more difficulties to overcome, cannot yet in any way be placed upon the same level; nevertheless, the progress which they have made in the last fifty years and the course which they are presently following, give us reason to hope that one day they will be able to bear comparison with the physical sciences. [288]

The object of this essay is to attempt to prove:

1. that the present manner of regarding the phenomena proper to living bodies is unsound in several respects; and

2. that these phenomena can all be explained in the same manner.

If I have been fortunate enough to have succeeded in my attempt and to have obtained the approval of the savants to whom I have the honor of presenting this paper, the physiological sciences will thus be brought closer to the physical sciences, at least in the course which they follow; and this will surely not be an indifferent advantage for them.

Let us first attempt to discover some of the reasons why the physiological sciences have remained backward.

Is it the facts which are lacking? Certainly not; for if it were possible for the quantity of facts to be a hindrance, this would certainly be the case in the physiological sciences.

Is it not rather the nature of these facts? That is more[289] probable: there can be no doubt that most of them seem inexact,[290] a situation which prevents the judicious savant from accepting them with confidence and drawing every possible advantage from them.

Finally, if we recall that it is often necessary to swallow a multitude of more or less absurd explanations and sometimes of supposed or ill-observed facts in order to reach any sure and significant data in the works on physiology, then we will easily appreciate that it is essential to have received unwearying patience and extremely sound judgement from nature to avoid being repelled by these tedious reasonings and led into error by these spurious or altered facts. This prompts us to think, along with certain persons whose opinions have the weight of authority, that most physiological facts need to be verified by new experiments, and that this is the sole means of rescuing the physics of living bodies from its present state of imperfection.

Another circumstance which contributes to retarding the progress of physiology is that the particular observations are not sufficiently generalized, and that the phenomena proper to organized bodies are not all related to one and the same cause, and finally that there is no uniform manner of explaining all these phenomena. We must not conceal the fact that the physiological sciences will never acquire the imposing certitude and perfection of the physical sciences so long as the defects just indicated are not remedied.

In accordance with this preliminary remark the course which I shall follow in this Memoir is naturally set out. We must first inquire whether the extremely varied phenomena which living bodies exhibit may not, in the final analysis, be highly multiplied modifications of some few phenomena which are observed in all organized beings throughout the entire duration of their existence, and which constitute their general and essential character. If we suppose this to be so, we must examine whether these general phenomena are of such a nature as to be related to a single cause, and whether they can all be subsumed under the same explanation.

Observation teaches that living bodies take from the substances in the midst of which they live, and carry to their interiors, a certain quantity of matter which generally bears the name of *nutritive matter* or *aliment*. Observation demonstrates that these same bodies allow to escape, in various forms, a more or less considerable quantity of the substance which immediately before served to compose them. These two facts, combined with certain others which are generally known, cause us correctly to admit as an assured fact that living bodies are not composed of the same matter at all stages of their existence; that, for example, after a certain interval of time, they are no longer formed of a single molecule of the substance which previously composed them. Thus it is now regarded as incontestable that all parts of a vegetable or an animal undergo a double intestine movement—one by which they are decomposed, that is to say, disencumbered of the matter which has become incapable of composing them any longer; and another by which they are recomposed, that is to say, they assimilate a certain proportion of new matter which will take on the vital properties and replace the losses which they have experienced through the movement of decomposition.

The series of intestine movements by which living bodies are decomposed and recomposed is designated by the physiologists with the name, nutrition. Nutrition must be considered one of the general phenomena which characterize organized bodies throughout the entire duration of their existence.

Since we have recognized a phenomenon common to all living beings, let us next see to what cause the physiologists relate it and what explanation they give of it.

The intestine movement which constitutes nutrition is not perceptible to our senses, and consequently its mode of action is entirely unknown to us; nevertheless, since we definitely see matter displaced, it becomes certain for us that there has been movement.

No analogy, not even a probable one, has yet been found between the play of ordinary chemical affinities and the nutritive movement; that is why this movement has always been considered—and still is today—as dependent upon a particular cause which, like planetary and molecular attraction, is unknown in its nature but manifest in its effects. This particular cause has received many denominations, but the best which has been given is that of *vital force*.

Up to this point our reasoning is perfect: we see phenomena which do not at all resemble the phenomena produced by attraction and which cannot be explained by it; thus we correctly suppose a particular cause for these phenomena.

The physiologists do not stop at this point. After having recognized a particular force as the cause of the nutritive movement, rather than ardently devoting themselves to the search for the laws of this force—a search which would be, without exception, the most beautiful and most interesting subject of work which anyone could propose for himself—they wish instead to see, in some fashion, how each molecule animated by the vital force acts in order to produce this nutritive movement; and thus they gratuitously suppose that the vital force is manifested in each molecule of a living body by two properties: the first, *sensibility* (the faculty of feeling, that is to say, of experiencing a more or less profound impression which changes the natural and usual rhythm of vibratility, etc.);[291] and the second, *motility* (the faculty of movement which consists in a continual tendency toward contraction or tightening, etc.).[292]

After having made this mere supposition the physiologists seem to forget that this is all that it is; at least they speak of these properties as if they really existed and as if they were established and verified by observation. I refer to the works of physiology in order to examine how nutrition is explained by means of sensibility and motility. Whatever explanation may be given in each of these works, it will be admitted that nothing in it is founded upon observation. What positive knowledge, then, do we have concerning nutrition?

Living bodies ordinarily lose a varied proportion of the matter which served to compose them for a longer or shorter time; these same bodies ordinarily take from outside themselves a variable quantity of matter upon which they act; this matter is soon transformed into their own substance, it composes them for a certain time, and afterwards abandons them. These two facts combined with the results of experiments on the coloring of bones[293] and some other analogous experiments, are all the positive knowledge we have concerning nutrition; and it is enough to cause the phenomenon to be recognized, but nothing more. To wish, after this, to explain nutrition by the supposition of vital properties; to wish to say, in some fashion, what the intestine—and probably very numerous—movements are by which these phenomena are effected; is, we must agree, to construct a mere hypothesis which is, in truth, very ingenious but which is none the less a pure supposition.

It seems to me that it would be worth just as much to limit ourselves to saying the following:

Nutrition is a phenomenon which cannot be reconciled with the phenomena observed in inert bodies; it is impossible, at the present time, to conceive that this phenomenon could be produced by the general laws of nature. There is no effect without a cause; hence nutrition depends upon a particular force which is unknown in its nature and manifested solely by its effects: this force is named the *vital force*.

Nevertheless, since a satisfying hypothesis is always useful to those who seek not to push back the limits of the science but only to profit from its advantages, I consent to what the physiologists admit concerning the vital properties bearing the names *sensibility* and *motility*. But the savant who has some idea of the means necessary for experimenting and for advancing the science ought not to delude himself about the true value of these expressions. What would be worth much more still than all these reasonings would be to perform experiments with a view to finding the general laws of the vital force. This labor is perhaps not as difficult as it is thought to be; and besides, even if it should be bristling with difficulties, its utility, should it succeed, and the honor of having undertaken it, should it not be followed with success, are more than determining reasons for undertaking it.[294]

A second phenomenon as general as *nutrition* is *action*.[295] In addition to the internal molecular movement which results in nutrition, there is exercised in each of the parts which compose a living body another molecular movement, just as invisible as the first and known, like it, simply by its results. For example, in animals of a superior order there exist parts called voluntary muscles which, under certain conditions, harden, shorten, and in a word, contract. This phenomenon is what is called an action: it depends upon an intimate movement carried out among the living molecules which together constitute the muscle.

Nearly all the parts of the animal body thus have, in addition to the nutritive movement, another internal movement the effect of which is called action. Thus the liver secretes bile, the salivary glands saliva, the testicles sperm, etc. These are facts recognized by everyone and they are all the more certain since they are susceptible to continual observation. In general, the more numerous and diversified are the actions of living bodies, the more perfect their life is said to be.[296]

Since actions are, for the most part, *appreciable* effects they do not give rise to any discussion; they are very thoroughly described; nothing is more firmly established than that muscles contract, the liver forms biles, the kidneys urine, etc. All would be well if we restricted outselves to sensible phenomena; but the mind of man is not of a nature to be contented with a fact, it absolutely must explain the fact and find a cause for it.[297] Now since observation can no longer guide anyone, each person adopts the opinion which most suits him; whence this character of things which are scarcely known or totally unknown being the inexhaustible subjects of disputations and discussions. This general remark is above all applicable to the action of living organs. In fact, what could be more disparate than the manner in which these actions are explained by the different authors? Mechanists, chemists, vitalists—all have supposed phenomena which they have carefully made to conform to their favorite opinions. For example, in how many different ways have they not explained, and are they not still explaining, the contraction of the voluntary muscles? The very supposition of a vital property, under the name of *voluntary contractility,* ought not, it seems to us, to be admitted; for it will presently be seen what must be thought about these vital properties which are particular to certain parts of an organized body.

Furthermore, this multitude of explanatory hypotheses, far from convincing and satisfying the true savant, causes him to appreciate all the more how necessary it is for him to devote himself to his researches.

Is it, then, so important to have an explanation of the insensible molecular movement from which action results? Who prevents us from repeating for action what we have said above for nutrition?

Action is a phenomenon proper to living beings; it does not at all resemble the phenomena observable in inorganic bodies: it seems to be the result of an intestine movement which takes place among the living molecules of the acting organ.

This molecular movement cannot, at this moment, be compared with those which occur within inert bodies. It is thus impossible to suppose that it depends upon the same cause; it is quite natural, on the contrary, to believe that it is governed by the same force which we have supposed, above, to preside over the nutritive movement. Accordingly, if we want an explanation we will prefer to choose the one which already serves to explain the nutritive movement, and we will explain action by the exercise of organic sensibility and of motility.

The physiologists presently follow this method for the explanation of the most frequent actions of the economy of living bodies, the *secretions.* It is generally agreed today that they are to be explained by the exercise of the two vital properties which I have just named.

If it were possible at this time to prove that all the phenomena of organized bodies can be related to nutrition or action, these phenomena could be regarded as produced by the same force, and they would be explained naturally in the same manner.

I am going to try to make this evident for the life of the animals of a superior order. The task will be so much the less difficult in that all the phenomena which together compose the life of the animal are already considered as produced by a particular force which has been recognized in all ages under diverse names, such as *physis, anima, vis, vita, impetum faciens, vital principle,* etc.

In accordance with what has preceded we have, in order to reach our goal, only to examine the phenomena which are not explained by *organic sensibility* and *insensible contractility*.

Before going any farther I hope I may be permitted to offer some general considerations on the action of organs.

Does each of the parts which compose an animal have a proper action? We can respond affirmatively for a great number of parts; we can say that it is probable for some of them; and we can respond negatively for many others.

There is, for example, no doubt that the muscle acts when it contracts, that the liver acts when it forms bile, that the heart acts when it expels blood from its cavities, that the brain acts when it perceives a sensation, etc.—these are parts whose actions are well-established. There are other parts whose actions are probable and simply supposed by analogy, or by the more powerful reason that nature has made nothing in vain: such parts are the thymus, the thyroid, the subrenal capsules, the lymphatic ganglia, and the nervous ganglia. Finally, there are many organs which appear to have no action, which seem entirely limited to the nutritive movement. The goal of nature was that these organs should exhibit, throughout the duration of their life, certain properties which are almost independent of the vital force: for example, the bones, the cartilage, the fibrous membranes, and several fluids such as those of the interior of the eye, the synovia, etc. In fact, these parts, in order to fulfill the role which is confided to them, need only present a certain form, a considerable resistance, and extremely tight connection between their molecules, a great deal of elasticity or of transparency, a disposition favorable to the refraction of light, etc.

Here a question of the highest importance presents itself. How does it happen that the actions of the living parts are so different from each other when they all depend upon one and the same cause?

I answer with one of the most general observations which it is possible to make concerning organized bodies. The nature, the disposition, and the mode of union of the living molecules—in a word, their organization—modify the vital force in such a way that the phenomena by which it is manifested in living bodies are always in a direct ratio to the organization of those bodies; so that I believe it is possible, even in the present state of the science, to establish that whenever the vital force animates a body of a given organization it will produce given phenomena.

Two living bodies with the same organization will exhibit the same vital phenomena; two living bodies organized differently will exhibit vital phenomena the diversity of which will always be in a direct ratio to the difference in organization.[298]

It is, in my opinion, extremely probable that if our means of investigating anatomical structures are developed in the future to a high degree of perfection, we will be able to account for the nuances of life as well as we now account for its great differences.[299] With what marvelous facility do the zoologists succeed in determining, in a rigorous manner, all the phenomena of the life of an animal, simply by considering one of its organs—a tarsal bone, for example! I consider this part of zoology to be one of the most remarkable and most satisfying things which has ever been accomplished.

I pass on, now to the consideration of the phenomena observed in the parts which, according to the physiologists, are endowed with particular vital properties.

It is, I believe, a great mistake to admit vital properties which are particular to some parts of organized bodies. Aside from the fact that this admission appears to me to be useless, it seems to me that a vital property ought to characterize life everywhere that the vital force has any influence; it ought to be common to all living bodies in the same way that extension, divisibility, impenetrability and mobility are the general properties of all bodies.

What do we mean and what, in fact, do we say when we admit a vital property which is particular to certain organs?—*sensible* organic contractility, for example: We say simply that the vital force is manifested in certain organs by a movement of contraction which is more or less varied according to the type of organ in question. Now because the vital force is characterized in one organ by a particular phenomenon, is it therefore necessary to create a vital property in order to explain it? But each organ presents different phenomena—by following this principle it would be necessary to multiply the vital properties to infinity and to create as many properties as there are different phenomena; it would be necessary to admit, after the example of the ancients and of some moderns, a digestive force, an assimilative force, a force of fixed situation, a force of vital resistance, etc.[300] If we suppose that the action of the heart depends upon a vital property, I see no reason why we do not also suppose that there exists in the liver a vital property which secretes bile and in the testicles one which forms sperm, etc. Perhaps someone will say to me that the intimate molecular movement necessary for the formation of bile or of sperm is not perceptible to our senses, and that it is thus a gratuitous supposition. I shall answer: Do we see any better what takes place in the interior of the heart at the time of its contraction? Is not this contraction the result of an intestine movement carried out among the living molecules which compose the heart?—a movement, furthermore, which has been generally recognized by the physiologists and which gave rise to many hypotheses when it was a question of explaining it.

In my opinion, the contraction of those organs which the authors endow with sensible organic contractility, is to those organs what bile is to the liver, and what sperm is to the testicles, etc. In order for the contraction to become apparent there must occur some sort of action among the parts composing those organs; in order for bile, sperm, etc., to be formed there must take place a series of molecular movements within the interior of the liver, the testicle, etc., the result of which is the formation of bile and of sperm.

If at this point someone wants to know why the intimate movement of the heart, etc., has as its effect a phenomenon called contraction, while the intimate movement of the liver, of the testicle, etc., has as its result the formation of bile, of sperm, etc., I shall recall the general observation and, if I dare employ the expression, the law of[301] the vital force which I noted above; namely: that the phenomena exhibited by a living body, or by one of its parts, are always in a direct ratio to its organization, so that the same organization entails the same vital phenomena while the least difference in this organization necessitates modification in these phenomena, etc.

Since the heart has an organization proper to distinct vital phenomena, and the liver and testicles have a completely different organization, these latter organs also have entirely different vital phenomena.

I conclude that the vital property known by the name of *sensible organic contractility, involuntary contractility,* etc., is nothing other than the action of the organs in which this property is supposed to exist. Since this action, like all the other actions, seems to be the effect of an intestine movement which takes place among the molecules of the organ, nothing prevents us from relating it to the vital force and explaining it by latent organic sensibility and by fibrillary contractility.

It still remains for me to examine those vital properties which are generally admitted under the names of *animal sensibility* or *sensiblity of relation,*[302] etc., and *animal contractility* or *voluntary contractility,* etc.

The reproach which I have just made against sensible organic contractility applies directly to these two properties as well; namely: thay they appertain only to certain parts of a limited number of organized bodies, and consequently they are not general and essential characters of life. In fact, I persist in thinking that if we admit vital properties—which, after all, it is not absolutely necessary to do—then we ought to conceive of them in such a way that they appertain to all organized and living beings.

I am prepared to admit, for the moment, that a vital property need not be common to all living bodies; but it ought, at least, to reside uniquely in the part in which it is supposed to exist, as do organic sensibility, fibrillary contractility, and sensible organic contractility. Let us see if animal sensibility and voluntary contractility possess this same character.

First, in what organs does *animal sensibility* reside? Does it reside in the external sense-organ? No, for if the nerve is cut or compressed, there is no sensation. In the nerve, then? No, for if the brain is diseased or compressed, again no sensation. Is it in the brain? No again, for if there is no sense-organ, or if the nerve is cut, there is no more sensation; if the brain is directly touched, it is insensible. Bichat certainly recognized this truth, for in his works and in his courses he considered animal sensibility (1st) in the sense-organ which receives, (2nd) in the nerve which transmits, and (3rd) in the brain which perceives the sensation.[303]

Thus there can be animal sensibility only insofar as there exists, in the same being, a sense-organ, a nerve and a brain. If one of these organs is lacking, or if it is slightly altered, there is no animal sensibility at all. What is a complex vital property?—I confess that I cannot conceive how authors of the greatest merit have failed to take this objection into account.

If, for the preceding reasons, we do not classify *animal sensibility* among the vital properties, how ought we to consider it? As a true function. A function is the common end of the action of a certain number of organs.

Digestion is the general result of the actions of the digestive organs; circulation is the general result of the actions of the circulatory organs; similarly, sensation is the general result of the actions of three organs; the sense-organ, the nerve and the brain. The eye acts in order to receive an impression, the optic nerve acts in order to transmit it and the brain acts in order to perceive it: the sum of these three actions is *sensation*. If, for any cause whatever, one of these actions does not take place there is no sensation; similarly, if the stomach or the liver, etc., does not act there is no digestion.

What we have just said with reference to animal sensibility must now be repeated for the contractility of the same name.

This pretended vital property does not reside in the muscle; for if the brain is compressed, no contraction; if the nerve is tied or cut, no contraction.

Bichat also considered animal contractility, first in the brain, then in the nerve, and finally in the muscle.[304] Voluntary contraction thus results from three actions; namely: the action of the brain,[305] the first cause of the contraction; the action of the nerve which transmits the cause of the contraction to[306] the muscle by which is produced the sensible phenomenon named contraction, the general effect of these three voluntary actions. If any one of these actions does not take place, no contraction.

Following this observation it is impossible not to consider animal contractility as a function which results from the actions of the brain, the nerve and the muscle.

Suppressing the two vital properties known by the names of animal sensibility and animal contractility, and considering them as functions instead, would be a most advantageous reform to accomplish in physiology; then there would be only a single manner of explaining the phenomena of life and the study of the science would be so much the easier.

When someone puts forward new ideas he must develop them as much as possible in order to make them evident to everyone; and this is why I want to show how sensation and voluntary contraction can be explained by organic sensibility and insensible contractility.

I begin with the sensations.

The sense-organs, like all active organs, have a double intestine movement. The first of these movements has nutrition as its end; while the second has as its result an action which is determined in relation to the organization of the organ, such as that of receiving an impression upon the occasion of contact with light, odors, vibrations of the air, etc. Light, for example, will strike in vain against the back of the eye if the retina is paralyzed; that is to say, if the retina cannot begin its action no impression will be produced or transmitted. It is thus necessary that the sense-organ act in order for an impression to be received; now for the very reason that the phenomena which a sense-organ exhibits can be related to actions in general, we have just shown that they are naturally explained by organic sensibility and insensible contractility. And the same can be said for the nerve: the nerve has its own organization; it is not surprising, then, that it should have a particular action—an action which consists in transmitting to the brain those impressions received from the sense-organ. This manner of regarding nervous transmission does away with the truly ridiculous supposition of a nervous fluid circulating through the nerves—a supposition which inadvertently recalls the infancy of physiology.[307]

As for what occurs in the brain at the moment of perception; it will be no innovation for me to say that it is an action. Almost all those who have, with some distinction, concerned themselves with the phenomena of intelligence have admitted an action of the brain at the moment when it perceives; and more recently Professor Chaussier has defined perception as *the action of the brain by which it grasps the impressions propagated from the sense-organs by the nerves.*[308]

I do not believe that it is necessary to repeat for animal contractility what I have just said for the sensibility of the same name.

It is clear that what is called animal contractility is nothing but a function which results from the action of three organs.[309]

Since each one of these three organs has a different texture, it also has a different action; and since an action is always preceded or accompanied by a molecular movement in the organ which acts, one ought in each case to relate this movement to the vital force and to explain it, if one judges this necessary, by organic sensibility and insensible contractility.

It thus becomes useless to admit a vital property under the name of animal contractility.

The physiologists have based their science upon an unsteady scaffolding, which perhaps explains why the physiological sciences are held in so little regard, sometimes even in the minds of those who cultivate them. But by bringing all the phenomena proper to living bodies into connection with nutrition and action—the first cause of which would be named vital force and would be supposed as manifesting itself through organic sensibility and insensible motility—we would permit that scaffolding to collapse of its own weight.

I conclude that all the phenomena proper to organized beings can be related to *nutrition* and to *action*, and that these two general phenomena are of such a nature as to be easily explained by organic sensibility and insensible contractility.

In closing I recall that these terms, *organic sensibility* and *fibrillary contractility,* designate no appreciable phenomena but only pure suppositions, simple manners of conceiving. It would perhaps be just as advantageous to commence the study of physiology at the instant when the phenomena of living bodies become appreciable to our senses. The part of the science which explains the intimate molecular movements of the organs is at this time, and will probably remain for a long time to come, nothing but a collection of conjectures which may be more or less related to the truth; it offers only a small number of useful applications and it always gives rise to discussions, the least inconvenience of which has been to cause the loss of time which ought to have been employed in performing experiments and in describing important phenomena with exactitude.

116 *William Randall Albury*

NOTES

1. C. Bernard, [Éloge de Magendie,] *Leçons sur les effets des substances toxiques et médicamenteuses* (Paris, 1857), pp. 1–37. Cf. C. Bernard, *De la physiologie générale* (Paris, 1872), pp. 5–10; J. T. Merz, *A History of European Thought in the Nineteenth Century* [1904–1912] (4v., New York, 1965), 2: 381–86; J. M. D. Olmsted, *François Magendie: Pioneer in Experimental Physiology and Scientific Medicine in XIX Century France* (New York, 1944), pp. 19–34; J. Schiller, *Claude Bernard et les problèmes scientifiques de son temps* (Paris, 1967), pp. 28–29, 44–49; and J. Schiller, *The Genesis and Structure of Claude Bernard's Experimental Method,* in *Foundations of Scientific Method: The Nineteenth Century,* ed. R. N. Giere and R. S. Westfall (Bloomington, Indiana, 1973), pp. 139–41. For a notable exception to the general tendency to follow Bernard's interpretation, see O. Temkin, *The philosophical background of Magendie's physiology,* Bull. Hist. Med. 20 (1946); 10–35, a paper which served, in many respects, as the starting point for the present study.
2. F. Magendie, *Essai sur les usages du voile du palais, avec quelques propositions sur la fracture du cartilage des côtes* (Paris, 1808), pp. 10–11. The quotations are taken from M.-F.-X. Bichat, *Traité d'anatomie descriptive* (5v., Paris, ans X–XII [1801–03]), 2: 403–4.
3. E.g., F. Magendie, *Précis élémentaire de physiologie* (2v., Paris, 1816–17), 1: 160; cf. J. M. D. Olmsted, *François Magendie,* p. 65.
4. M.-F.-X. Bichat, *Recherches physiologiques sur la vie et la mort,* ed. F. Magendie (4e éd., Paris, 1822); *Traité des membranes en général et de diverses membranes en particulier,* ed. F. Magendie (2e éd., Paris, 1827); and *Recherches physiologiques,* ed. F. Magendie (5e éd., Paris, 1829). The quotation is taken from Magendie's preface to the 1822 edition of the *Recherches physiologiques.* (All translations in this study are my own unless otherwise indicated.)
5. The first memoir was divided into two parts, one of which was read by Magendie at the end of April and the other by Delille some time in May. The text of this memoir was never published, although two summaries, each dealing with the entire memoir, appeared in contemporary journals: see F. Magendie and R. Delille, *Extrait d'un Mémoire ayant pour titre: Examen de l'action de quelques végétaux sur la moelle épinière; lu à l'Institut de France, le 24 avril 1809, par M. Magendie, docteur en médecine,* Bull. des sci. méd. de la Soc. méd. d'émulation de Paris 3 (1809): 411–16; and *Des effets de l'Upas Tienté* [sic] *sur l'économie animale; par MM. Delille et Magendie: Institut Nat., Mai 1809,* Nouv. bull, des sci. par la Soc. philomath. de Paris 1 (1807–09): 368–71. The second memoir, read entirely by Magendie, was also summarized in a contemporary periodical and later published in full in Magendie's own journal: *Nouvelles expériences avec l'Upas Tieuté; par MM. Magendie et Delille: Institut Nat.,* Nouv. bull. des sci. par la Soc. philomath. de Paris 1 (1807–09): 404–6; and *Mémoire sur les organes de l'absorption chez les mammifères; lu à l'Institut, le 7 août 1809, par M. Magendie, docteur en médecine,* J. de physiol. exp. et path. 1 (1821): 18–32. The third memoir was read entirely by Delille: *Examen des effets de l'upas antiar et de plusieurs substances émétiques* [lu le 28 août 1809], Procès-verb. de l'Acad. des sci. 4 (1809): 242, 275.
6. C. Bernard, *Leçons de physiologie opératoire* (Paris, 1879), p. 335.
7. F. Magendie and R. Delille, *Mémoire sur les organes d'absorption,* p. 18n.
8. C. Bernard, *Physiologie opératoire,* p. 335. For a discussion of eighteenth-century ideas on the absorbent function of the lymphatic system, see N. B. Eales, *The history of the lymphatic system, with special reference to the Hunter-Monro controversy,* J. Hist. Med. 29 (1974): 280–94.
9. C. Bernard, *Physiologie opératoire,* p. 335.
10. For an application of this concept of ''structural similarity'' to the procedures of Galen and Harvey, see O. Temkin, *A Galenic model for quantitative physiological reasoning?* Bull. Hist. Med. 35 (1961): 470–75. It was Dr. Temkin who first suggested to me, in the course of an informal conversation, that I look carefully at Bichat's experiments.
11. F. Magendie and R. Delille, *Examen de l'action de quelques végétaux* and *Des effets de l'Upas Tienté,* passim.
12. F. Magendie and R. Delille, *Mémoire sur les organes de l'absorption,* p. 19.
13. Ibid., pp. 21–22. (On Dupuytren, see reference 309, below.)
14. Ibid., p. 23.

15. Ibid., pp. 23–24.

16. This demonstration was singled out by Georges Cuvier for special mention in his 1808 report to Napoleon on the nonmathematical sciences: "On doutoit du lieu précis où ce changement s'opère. Des expériences très-ingénieuses de Bichat ont prouvé que c'est au passage même des artères dans les veines pulmonaires et d'une manière subite que le sang devient rouge." G. Cuvier, *Rapport historique sur les progrès des sciences naturelles depuis 1789, et sur leur état actuel* (Paris, 1810), p. 239.

17. M.-F.-X. Bichat, *Recherches physiologiques* (1e éd., Paris, an VIII [1800]), p. 299. (This edition used in all subsequent references to this work.) Earlier experiments had been carried out on this subject by the English physician Richard Lower (1631–92); see R. Lower, *Tractatus de Corde. Item de motu et colore sanguinis et chyli in eum Transitu* [1669], reprinted with introduction and translation by K. J. Franklin in *Early Science in Oxford*, ed. R. T. Gunther (Oxford, 1932), v. 9.

18. M.-F.-X. Bichat, *Recherches physiologiques*, pp. 302–4.

19. In his *Recherches physiologiques* Bichat attempted to maintain neutrality on the question of whether the reddening of blood resulted from the entry of oxygen into the blood or from the discharge by the blood of hydrogen and carbon into the oxygen in the lungs.—e.g., p. 305. But he sometimes seemed to favor the first of these alternatives, as when he spoke of "le principe qui sert à cette coloration [passant] directement du poumon dans le sang."—p. 307. Similarly, in later works he referred to pulmonary vessels "qui prennent dans l'air les substances propres à colorer le sang." *Anatomie générale, appliquée à la physiologie et à la médecine* (4v., Paris, an X [1801]), 2: p. 626. At any rate, by the time of Magendie's researches on absorption, Bichat's experiment was interpreted as a demonstration of "l'action de l'oxigène sur du sang." G. Cuvier, *Rapport historique*, p. 239.

20. M.-F.-X. Bichat, *Recherches physiologiques*, p. 307.

21. F. Magendie and R. Delille, *Examen de l'action de quelques végétaux*, p. 413; and *Des effets de l'Upas Tienté*, p. 369.

22. G. Cuvier, *Rapport historique*, p. 240.

23. F. Magendie and R. Delille, *Mémoire sur les organes de l'absorption*, p. 24.

24. Ibid., p. 25.

25. Ibid., pp. 25–26.

26. M.-F.-X. Bichat, *Traité des membranes* (1e éd., Paris, an VIII [1799]). (This edition used in all subsequent references to this work.)

27. M.-F.-X. Bichat, *Recherches physiologiques*, pp. 195–96.

28. M.-F.-X. Bichat, *Traité des membranes*, pp. 68–69.

29. Ibid., pp. 69–71.

30. Ibid., p. 71.

31. Ibid., pp. 71–72.

32. F. Magendie and R. Delille, *Mémoire sur les organes de l'absorption*, pp. 26–27.

33. Ibid., p. 27.

34. Ibid., pp. 27–28.

35. Ibid., p. 32.

36. Ibid., p. 28.

37. Ibid., p. 29.

38. Ibid., p. 30.

39. Ibid., p. 31.

40. Ibid., p. 32. Claude Bernard, in repeating Magnedie's transfusion experiments, explained why the animals receiving the toxic blood had failed to develop the signs of poisoning, by pointing out that Magendie had not prolonged the transfusion sufficiently to allow an accumulation of *upas* in the recipient animal to the level necessary to produce the characteristic convulsions. Since the transfused blood was being added to the recipient's normal quantity of blood it would take longer for an effective level of concentration to be reached. C. Bernard, *Physiologie opératoire*, p. 339; cf. J. M. D. Olmsted, *François Magendie*, pp. 40–41.

41. M.-F.-X. Bichat, *Recherches physiologiques*, pp. 250–51. Here Bichat was opposing the view of Edmund Goodwyn (1755–1829), who held that the black blood failed to stimulate the

arterial side of the heart, which consequently ceased beating. It was only as a result of the cessation of the circulation, Goodwyn maintained, that unconsciousness occurred in cases of asphyxiation. See E. Goodwyn, *The Connexion of Life with Respiration* (London, 1789); French translation by J. N. Hallé published in Mag. encyclopédique 1[4] (1795): 438–70 and 1[5] (1795): 32–78.

42. M.-F.-X. Bichat, *Recherches physiologiques,* pp. 280–82.

43. Ibid., pp. 283–84.

44. Ibid., p. 285.

45. Ibid., pp. 285–87; cf. Bichat's "control" transfusion, using normal arterial blood only, ibid., p. 279.

46. Ibid., pp. 327–28.

47. It should be clearly noted that in drawing this conclusion we do not claim to have shown that Magendie necessarily "borrowed" his experimental procedures directly from Bichat, or that he was somehow "influenced" by Bichat's experimental technique. Most of the individual operations involved in the experiments we have examined were practiced by other physiologists before and after Bichat, so it is not the origin and transmission of these operations that concerns us. Rather, our concern is with the systematic combination of these operations to investigate a particular vital phenomenon, and with the pattern of reasoning revealed by that combination. Whether Magendie designed his own experiments completely in isolation from Bichat's work, or whether (as seems probable) he intentionally or unintentionally adapted Bichat's experiments to new physiological circumstances, the effect was the same: that Magendie's investigation of the process of absorption was carried out by means of a series of experiments that systematically paralleled the ones that Bichat had used to study the phenomena of respiration. In the second part of this study we shall discuss the theoretical conditions that made this parallelism possible.

48. C. Bernard, *Éloge de Magendie,* p. 10.

49. ". . . le plus important des collaborateurs médicaux de l'*Encyclopédie* est un homme dont on a peu parlé, le docteur Ménuret de Chambaud, qui rédigea plus de quarante articles dans les dix derniers tomes, et fit du grand dictionnaire l'instrument d'une propagande passionnée en faveur d'une doctrine révolutionnaire, celle de la nouvelle école de Montpellier, dont Bordeu lui-même n'est en somme que le plus célèbre représentant.'' J. Roger, *Les sciences de la vie dans la pensée française du XVIIIe siècle* (Paris, 1963), p. 631.

50. J.-J. Ménuret de Chambaud, *Observateur,* Encyclopédie, ou Dictionnaire raisonné des sciences, des arts et des métiers, ed. D. Diderot and J. L. d'Alembert (2e éd., 30v., Genève, 1777–79), 23: 287B.

51. J.-J. Ménuret de Chambaud, *Observation,* ibid., pp. 294B, 295A, 295B–296A.

52. A. von Haller, *A Dissertation on the Sensible and Irritable Parts of Animals* [1775], trans. anonymous, ed. O. Temkin (Baltimore, 1936), p. 7.

53. Ibid., p. 8.

54. Ibid., p. 16.

55. Ibid.; cf. p. 12.

56. Ibid., p. 47.

57. Quoted in J. Roger, *Les sciences de la vie,* p. 635.

58. Bordeu, for example, "se classe parmi les médecins 'naturistes', 'observateurs', 'exspectateurs', qui se contentent de suivre, et de faciliter parfois avec prudence, l'action de 'ce qu'on appelle la nature', c'est-à-dire, de ce 'principe particulier qui veille sans cesse à la conservation des corps'.'' Ibid., p. 629, with quotations from Bordeu's *Recherches sur l'histoire de la médecine* (1768). The concept of the healing force of nature was not, of course, a new development of the Montpellier school, but was derived from Hippocratic medicine.

59. J.-J. Ménuret de Chambaud, *Observation,* p. 293B.

60. "But the theory why some parts of the human body are endowed with these [vital] properties, while others are not, I shall not at all meddle with. For I am persuaded that the source of both lies concealed beyond the reach of the knife and microscope, beyond which I do not chuse to hazard many conjectures, as I have no desire of teaching what I am ignorant of myself.'' A. von Haller, *Dissertation,* p. 8.

61. M.-F.-X. Bichat, *Recherches physiologiques,* p. ii.

62. M.-F.-X. Bichat, *Discourse on the study of physiology* [1798]. See appendix herein, pp. 97–115. (For the date of this lecture, see A. Arène, *Essai sur la philosophie de Xavier Bichat*. Arch. d'anthropol. crim. 26 (1911): 763.

63. Ibid.

64. Ibid.

65. Ibid.

66. Ibid.

67. Ibid.

68. Ibid.

69. See J. M. D. Olmsted, *François Magendie*, pp. 26–27.

70. M.-F.-X. Bichat, *Discourse*.

71. M.-F.-X. Bichat, *Recherches physiologiques*, p. 94.

72. Ibid., pp. 94–95.

73. Ibid., p. 105.

74. Ibid., p. 257.

75. M.-F.-X. Bichat, *Discourse*.

76. Ibid.; cf. *Anatomie général*, 1: 1v.

77. M.-F.-X. Bichat, *Discourse*.

78. O. Temkin, *Philosophical background*, p. 29n.

79. M.-F.-X. Bichat, *Anatomie générale*, 1: vii. We may note that Bichat continues this passage with the following proposition, "que tout phénomène thérapeutique a pour principe leur retour au type naturel dont elles étoient écartées."—Ibid. The contrast between Bichat's position on medical treatment and the therapeutic nihilism of the Montpellier school arises from the more fundamental contrast between Bichat's largely deterministic conception of vital phenomena and the Montpellier school's emphasis on the spontaneity of life (see reference 58, above).

80. See the discussion in the section entitled "Bichat's System of Vital Properties," herein.

81. M.-F.-X. Bichat, *Discourse*.

82. M.-F.-X. Bichat, *Traité des membranes*, pp. 73–74.

83. Ibid., p. 143.

84. Ibid., p. 142.

85. M.-F.-X. Bichat, *Recherches physiologiques*, p. 192.

86. Cf. O. Temkin, *Materialism in French and German physiology of the early nineteenth century*, Bull. Hist. Med. 20 (1946): 322: "Whether vital properties were believed to counteract the physical and chemical processes [Bichat] or whether a vital force was assumed to cover our ignorance regarding nutrition and so-called vital actions [Magendie], the result was the same in so far as the laws of inanimate nature were declared insufficient to explain all the manifestations of life."

87. M.-F.-X. Bichat, *Discourse*.

88. F. Magendie, *An Elementary Summary of Physiology*, trans. J. S. Forsyth (2v., London, 1825) 1: ix (an English translation of the *Précis élémentaire*).

89. M.-F.-X. Bichat, *Discourse*.

90. Cf. the rules which Bichat drew up for the *Société médicale d'émulation* in 1796:

"VI. L'observation étant la première base des sciences naturelles, chaque membre s'engage à recueillir et à communiquer à la société tous les faits intéressans qui s'offriront à ses recherches.

"VII. Á l'observation s'unit l'expérience; de là une seconde branche de travail renfermant les expériences anciennes à repeter, et les nouvelles à entreprendre." [M.-F.-X. Bichat] *Reglemens de la Société médicale d'émulation*, Mag. encyclopédique 2[3] (1796): 262. On Bichat's authorship of these rules, see A. F. T. Levacher de la Feutrie, *Éloge de Marie-François-Xavier Bichat*, Mém. de la Soc. méd. d'émulation 5 (1803): xlii.

91. M.-F.-X. Bichat, *Anatomie générale*, 1: xxxix.

92. M.-F.-X. Bichat, *Recherches physiologiques*, p. 1.

93. M.-F.-X. Bichat, *Discourse*. (Cf. *Recherches physiologiques*, pp. 2–4.)

94. Ibid.

95. "Lorsque les faits observés dans l'état de santé semblent se taire et ne rien décider en faveur de son opinion, il [Bichat] a recours, avec son intelligence ordinaire, aux observations

faites dans l'état de maladie, et persuade." G. L. Duvernoy, *Recherches physiologiques sur la vie et la mort, par Xavier Bichat,* Mag. encyclopédique 6[3] (1800): 309.

96. M.-F.-X. Bichat, *Recherches physiologiques,* p. 102.

97. Ibid., p. 191. By contrast with the first part of Bichat's *Recherches,* wrote Duvernoy in his review, the second part "est absolument expérimentale." G. L. Duvernoy, *Recherches physiologiques... par Xavier Bichat,* p. 321.

98. M.-F.-X. Bichat, *Mémoire sur la membrane synoviale des articulations,* Mém. de la Soc. mèd. d'émulation 2 (1799): 350–70. This memoir contains only one experiment, p. 356. which was undertaken to confirm a pathological observation.

99. M.-F.-X. Bichat, *Discourse.*

100. Ibid.

101. Ibid.

102. See, for example, M.-F.-X. Bichat, *Traité des membranes,* p. 32.

103. F. Magendie, *Quelques idées générales sur les phénomènes particuliers aux corps vivans,* Bull, des sci. méd. de la Soc. méd. d'émulation de Paris 4 (1809): 147. [*Some general ideas on the phenomena peculiar to living bodies.* (See appendix herein, pp. 107–115.)]

104. O. Temkin, *Philosophical background,* p. 35.

105. C. Bernard, *Éloge de Magendie,* p. 10.

106. F. Magendie and R. Delille, *Des effets de l'Upas Tienté,* p. 370.

107. M.-F.-X. Bichat, *Traité des membranes,* p. 68.

108. M.-F.-X. Bichat, *Anatomie générale* 2: 412. The term "venous absorption" does not appear in Bichat's text, but in the table of contents only.

109. "I call that part of the human body irritable, which becomes shorter upon being touched; very irritable if it contracts upon a slight touch, and the contrary if by a violent touch it contracts but little.

"I call that a sensible part of the human body, which upon being touched transmits the impression of it to the soul; and in brutes, in whom the existence of a soul is not so clear, I call those parts sensible, the irritation of which occasions evident signs of pain and disquiet in the animal. On the contrary, I call that insensible, which being burnt, tore, pricked, or cut till it is quite destroyed, occasions no sign of pain nor convulsion, nor any sort of change in the situation of the body....

"We see that experiments only can enable us to define what parts of the human body are sensible or irritable, and what the physiologists and physicians have said upon these qualities, without having made experiments, has been the source of a great many errors, both in this case and in a number of others." A. von Haller, *Dissertation,* pp. 8–9.

110. C. Bernard, *Éloge de Magendie,* p. 10.

111. F. Magendie, *Elementary Summary,* 1: vii–viii.

112. O. Temkin, *Philosophical background,* p. 32.

113. Cf. G. Rosen, *The philosophy of ideology and the emergence of modern medicine in France,* Bull. Hist. Med. 20 (1946): 328–39.

114. F. Magendie, *Elementary Summary,* 1: ix.

115. O. Temkin, *Philosophical background,* p. 33.

116. Ibid., p. 34.

117. F. Magendie, *Elementary Summary,* 1: viii.

118. F. Magendie, *Some general ideas.*

119. J. Schiller, *Claude Bernard,* p. 44; cf. *Physiology's struggle for independence in the first half of the nineteenth century,* Hist. of Sci. 7 (1968): 65.

120. F. Magendie, *Some general ideas.*

121. Ibid.

122. M.-F.-X. Bichat, *Recherches physiologiques,* pp. 98–121.

123. M.-F.-X. Bichat, *Anatomie générale,* 1: lxxxii–lxxxiii.

124. Ibid., pp. 5–6.

125. Ibid., pp. vii, lxxxii–lxxxv.

126. C. Bernard, *Éloge de Magendie,* p. 7.

127. J. M. D. Olmsted, *François Magendie,* p. 31.

128. F. Magendie, *Some general ideas.*

129. P.-J. Barthez, *Nouveaux éléments de la science de l'homme* (2e éd., 2v., Paris, 1806), 1: 112.

130. Ibid., p. 116.

131. Ibid., p. 114.

132. Ibid., p. 131.

133. Ibid., p. 117.

134. Ibid., p. 181.

135. F. Chaussier, *Table synoptique des propriétés charactéristiques et des principaux phénomènes de la force vitale* (Paris, s.d.); cf. the quotations from this work in references 291, 292, and 294, below.

136. C. L. Dumas, *Principes de physiologie* (2e éd., 4v., Paris, 1806), 1: 116.

137. Ibid., p. 119.

138. Ibid., p. 122.

139. Ibid., p. 129.

140. Ibid., p. 130.

141. Ibid., pp. 131–32.

142. B.-A. Richerand, *Nouveaux élémens de physiologie* (2e éd., 2v., Paris, an X [1802]), 1: lvi. Despite the similarities of their systems, Richerand was a critic rather than a follower of Bichat; see B.-A. Richerand, *Réflexions critiques sur un ouvrage ayant pour titre, Traité des Membranes, par le C. Bichat*, Mag. encyclopédique 5[6] (1799): 289–306.

143. Cf. the remarks in G. Cuvier, *Rapport historique*, pp. 218, 219, 231, 233, 239, 240, 241, 339, 342, and 362.

144. F. Magendie, *Some general ideas*.

145. Ibid.

146. Ibid.

147. Ibid.

148. Ibid.

149. Ibid.

150. Ibid.

151. Ibid.

152. Ibid.

153. Ibid.

154. Ibid.

155. Ibid.

156. Ibid.

157. Ibid.

158. Ibid.

159. Ibid.

160. Ibid.

161. Ibid.

162. Ibid.

163. Ibid.

164. F. Magendie, *Elementary Summary*, 1: 13.

165. F. Magendie, *Some general ideas*.

166. See B.-A. Richerand, *Essai sur la connexion de la vie avec la circulation*, Mém. de la Soc. méd. d'émulation 3 (1800): 296–310, and *Note sur la susceptibilité galvanique, dans les Animaux à sang chaud*, Mém. de la Soc. méd. d'émulation 3 (1800): 311 ff. On Chaussier, see G. Cuvier, *Rapport historique*, pp. 240–41, and reference 309, below.

167. F. Magendie, *Some general ideas*.

168. Ibid.

169. O. Temkin, *The classical roots of Glisson's doctrine of Irritation*, Bull. Hist. Med. 38 (1964): 297–306; cf. T. S. Hall, *On biological analogs of Newtonian paradigms*, Phil. of Sci. 35 (1968): 11–12, and *Ideas of Life and Matter* (2v., Chicago, 1969), 1: 396–97.

170. O. Temkin, *Classical roots*, p. 306.

171. Quoted in ibid., p. 298n.; cf. Haller's remarks quoted in H. Marion, *Francis Glisson*, Rev. phil. 14 (1882): 126–27.

172. O. Temkin, *Introduction* in A. von Haller, *Dissertation,* p. 2.

173. See the account in J. Roger, *Les sciences de la vie,* pp. 618–41, and our section on "Methodological background," above.

174. See, for example, É. B. de Condillac, *La logique* [1780], esp. Part I, chapter 2, in *Oeuvres philosophiques de Condillac,* ed. G. LeRoy (3v., Paris, 1947–1951), 2: 374–76, and my Ph.D. dissertation, *The Logic of Condillac and the Structure of French Chemical and Biological Theory, 1780–1801,* Johns Hopkins Univ., 1972 (a translation of the former work and a revision of the latter are currently being prepared for publication). My conclusions on the epistemology of the classical period agree substantially with those presented in M. Foucault, *The Order of Things,* trans. anonymous (New York, 1970), chapter 3.

175. É. B. de Condillac, *Oeuvres philosophiques* 1: 1–118 and 219–317.

176. Théophile de Bordeu, *Recherches anatomiques sur la position des glandes et sur leur action* (Paris, 1751), p. 373.

177. J. Roger, *Les sciences de la vie,* p. 635; cf. J.-J. Ménuret de Chambaud, *Oeconomie Animale,* Encyclopédie, ed. D. Diderot and J. L. d'Alembert (2e éd., 30 v., Genève, 1777–79), 23: 418B.

178. P.-J. Barthez, *Nouveaux éléments,* 1: 203.

179. P.-J.-G. Cabanis, *Oeuvres philosophiques de Cabanis,* ed. C. Lehec and J. Cazeneuve (2 v., Paris, 1956), 1: 165.

180. T. S. Hall, *Biological analogs.*

181. C. L. Dumas, *Principes,* 1: 117.

182. P.-J.-G. Cabanis, *Oeuvres phiolosophiques,* 1: 531–32; cf. O. Temkin, *Philosophical background,* pp. 20–21.

183. M.-F.-X. Bichat, *Anatomie générale,* 1: xxxvii.

184. F. Magendie, *Elementary Summary,* 1: 11. It will be recalled that Magendie also referred to a vital force which he compared to physical and chemical forces; however, two important distinctions must be noted in relation to this point: (1) for Magendie the comparison was drawn only at the epistemological level (each force being "unknown in its nature but manifest in its effects") and was never extended to the ontological level; and (2) the vital force, according to Magendie, gave rise to no macroscopic phenomena, but only to imperceptible molecular motions that could not be investigated directly; thus the vital force was not the direct object of study for Magendie, who recommended that physiologists concern themselves with "the phenomena of living bodies [which are] appreciable to our senses." See our section on "Magendie's explanatory system," above.

185. See E. B. de Condillac, *La logique,* Part 2, *Oeuvres philosophiques,* 2: 393–414; cf. M. Foucault, *The Order of Things,* pp. 71–76.

186. See, for example, M.-F.-X. Bichat, *Anatomie générale,* 1: vii–viii and xxxix–xl.

187. H. Daudin, *Cuvier et Lamarck. Les classes zoologiques et l'idée de série animale* (2 v., Paris, 1926), chapters 1, 8, and 9; W. Coleman, *Georges Cuvier, Zoologist* (Cambridge, Mass., 1964), chapter 2; and M. Foucault, *The Order of Things,* pp. 263–74. One interesting indication of the epistemological distance between Cuvier and physiologists such as Bichat may be found in Cuvier's attitude toward analysis and synthesis in his "Discours d'ouverture" of 1795. While acknowledging the importance of analysis as a method of discovery, Cuvier held that a science, once constituted, could be adequealty taught by the synthetic method of beginning with general principles and descending to particulars. (See G. Cuvier, *Discours prononcé par le citoyen Cuvier, à l'ouverture du cours d'Anatomie comparée qu'il fait au Muséum national d'histoire naturelle pour le citoyen Mertrud,* Mag. encyclopédique 1[5] [1795]: 149–51.) For Bichat, on the contrary, it was only the analytic method that could lead the student to a proper comprehension of any science.

188. C. Bernard, *Éloge de Magendie,* p. 30.

189. J. Schiller, *Genesis and structure,* p. 134.

190. G. Cuvier, *Leçons d'anatomie comparée* (5 v., Paris, 1800–05), 1: v.

191. Ibid.; cf. W. Coleman, *Georges Cuvier,* p. 63.

192. G. Canguilhem, *La formation du concept de réflexe aux XVIIe et XVIIIe siècles* (Paris, 1955), p. 90.

193. M. Gross, *Cuvier and a Transformation in Physiology in France*. (paper read at the Joint Atlantic Seminar in the History of Biology, Boston, Mass., April 7, 1973); and R. M. Young, *Mind, Brain and Adaptation* (Oxford, 1970), pp. 57–60. Cuvier's unpublished lectures of 1807 and 1809 were devoted to the nervous and muscular systems, and acknowledged the value of experimentation in investigating the functioning of these systems. W. Coleman, *Georges Cuvier*, pp. 36–37 and 90–91; cf. reference 287, below.

194. See, for example, Cuvier's endorsement of Kant's dictum that "la raison de la manière d'être de chaque partie d'un corps vivant réside dans l'ensemble." G. Cuvier, *Anatomie comparée*, 1: 6.

195. Cf. Claude Perrault's programmatic statement of 1667 for the *Académie royale des sciences:* "à chaque organe trouver sa fonction, pour chaque fonction trouver l'organe." Quoted in J. Schiller, *Claude Bernard*, p. 26.

196. G. Cuvier, *Anatomie comparée*, 1: 34–35.

197. Ibid., pp. 63–64.

198. F. Magendie, *Some general ideas*. Schiller has interpreted this definition as a "nouvelle conception de la fonction introduite par Magendie en 1809 et qui répresente une rupture avec le passé." J. Schiller, *Physiologie et classification dans l'oeuvre de Lamarck*, Hist. et biol. 2 (1969): 46; cf. *Claude Bernard*, pp. 28, 47.

199. M.-F.-X. Bichat, *Leçons de physiologie*—an X (MS. lecture notes of L. N. Jusserandot, collection of the Medezinhistorisches Institut der Universität Zürich), p. [3]. My attention was drawn to the Jusserandot manuscripts by the references in E. H. Ackerknecht, *Medicine at the Paris Hospital, 1794–1848* (Baltimore, 1967), pp. 56 and 131. I wish to thank the director of the Zurich Institute, Prof. H. Koelbing, for having made available to me a microfilm copy of portions of these manuscripts.

200. M.-F.-X. Bichat, *Anatomie descriptive*, 1: xi and xix.

201. Ibid., p. xv.

202. See, for example, the table in Bichat's 1798 *Discourse*.

203. F. Magendie, *Elementary Summary*, 1: 17.

204. F. Vicq-d'Azyr, *Oeuvres recueillies de Vicq-d'Azyr*, ed. J.-L. Moreau de la Sarthe (6 v., Paris, 1805), v. 4; cf. reference 241, below. It is reported that Bichat's library "contenait tous les bons ouvrages, et surtout ceux de Haller et de Vicq-d'Azyr." H. M. D. de Blainville, *Histoire des sciences de l'organisation et de leurs progrès, comme base de la philosophie*, ed. F. L. M. Maupied (3 v., Paris et Lyon, 1845), 3: 185.

205. T. de Bordeu, *Recherches anatomiques*, pp. 451–52.

206. M.-F.-X. Bichat, *Anatomie générale*, 1: lxxix–lxxx.

207. M.-F.-X. Bichat, *Anatomie descriptive*, 1: xiv.

208. F. Magendie, *Elementary Summary*, 1: 16–17.

209. A striking example of Magendie's insistence upon experimental investigation rather than anatomical deduction may be found in his earliest published references to Claude Bernard. In his 1839 lectures on the nervous system Magendie twice had Bernard prepare dissections of the facial nerves of a rabbit, the first time to demonstrate the path of a nerve *after* experiments had been carried out on its function, and the second time to show that despite the extreme care taken in the dissection, the function of the nerve in question could only be determined experimentally: "La question est très difficile à résoudre par l'anatomie.... Il faudra, je le répète, de nouvelles expériences." F. Magendie, *Leçons sur les fonctions et les maladies du système nerveux* (2 v., Paris, 1839), 2: 181–82 and 207–8; cf. J. M. D. Olmsted and E. H. Olmsted, *Claude Bernard and the Experimental Method in Medicine* (New York, 1952), p. 24. Earlier in the same series of lectures Magendie conceded that perhaps something could be learned about the function of the arteries from an examination of their structure, however he denied that anything of the kind was possible with the nerves: "Mais le nerf, que savez-vous de ses usages par l'examen de son tissu?... Rien n'indique qu'il ait telle fonction plutôt que telle autre.... Vous le piquez, et l'animal manifeste de la souffrance. Voilà que nous commençons à être sur la voie de ses usages; mais alors remarquez qu'il n'est plus question de scalpel ni de dissections minutieuses: vous êtes sur le terrain de la physiologie expérimentale." (F. Magendie, *Les fonctions et les maladies*, 2: 6.)

210. Cf. J. Schiller, *Physiology's struggle*, p. 74, and *Genesis and structure*, p. 151. For an illuminating discussion of the differences between Magendie's "physiological" approach and Sir Charles Bell's "anatomical" approach to the functions of the spinal nerve roots, see J. M. D. Olmsted, *François Magendie*, chapter 7. In contrast to Magendie, Bell believed that "inference from anatomical fact is the royal road to discovery" in physiology. L. Stevenson, *Anatomical reasoning in physiological thought*, in *The Historical Development of Physiological Thought*, ed. C. McC. Brooks and P. F. Cranefield (New York, 1959), p. 33.

211. Cf. J. Schiller, *Claude Bernard*, p. 28.

212. Cf. the remarks of M. D. Grmek and G. Canguilhem, in F. Courtès, *Georges Cuvier ou l'origine de la négation*, Rev. d'hist. des sci. 23 (1970): 31–32; and M. Foucault, *La situation de Cuvier dans l'histoire de biologie—II*, Rev. d'hist. des sci. 23 (1970): 73–74.

213. F. Magendie, *Mémoire sur le méchanisme de l'absorption chez les animaux à sang rouge et chaud*, J. de physiol. exp. et path. 1 (1821): 2. The same kind of analogy can be found in the works of Cuvier, e.g.: "outre que l'absorption des matières alimentaires, . . . il y a une autre absorption qui se fait continuellement à la surface extérieure, et une troisième qui a lieu par l'effet de la respiration." G. Cuvier, *Anatomie comparée*, 1: 4.

214. M.-F.-X. Bichat, *Anatomie générale*, 2: 626.

215. In other words, the "answers" provided by the older theoretical problematic became "questions" within the new one. See the discussion of "l'emploi raisonnable de terme de *forces vitales*," in G. Cuvier, *Rapport historique*, pp. 224 ff., and Cuvier's remarks *On the Use of the Vital Principle in Physiology* in the appendix, below. So different was Magendie's understanding of "sensibility" and "contractility" from that of his predecessors that while criticizing their use of these terms he was forced to write: "I confess that I cannot conceive how authors of the greatest merit have failed to take this objection into account." F. Magendie, *Some general ideas*.

216. G. Cuvier, *Rapport historique*, p. 231; cf. pp. 227–28: "c'est par un abus de mots, qu'on en étend la dénomination aux fonctions de ce système [nerveux] qui ne sont point accompagnées de perception."

217. Ibid., p. 200.

218. Ibid., p. 201.

219. F. Magendie, *Some general ideas*.

220. G. Cuvier, *Rapport historique*, pp. 225 and 228–30.

221. F. Magendie, *Some general ideas*.

222. Ibid.

223. Ibid.

224. G. Cuvier, *Rapport historique*, p. 330; cf. W. Coleman, *Georges Cuvier*, pp. 67–72.

225. G. Cuvier, *Anatomie comparée*, 1: 4; cf. M. Foucault, *La situation de Cuvier*, pp. 68 and 84; and C. Limoges *L'économie naturelle et le principe de corrélation chez Cuvier et Darwin*, Rev. d'hist. des sci. 23 (1970): 40.

226. F. Magendie, *Elementary Summary*, 1: 15–16.

227. Cf. F. L. Holmes, *Origins of the concept of the milieu intérieur*, in *Claude Bernard and Experimental Medicine*, ed. F. Grande and M. B. Visscher (Cambridge, Mass., 1967), p. 180.

228. F. Magendie, *Elementary Summary*, 1: viii–ix and 11. In terms of this comparison with physics we would hold that Magendie was the Galileo of physiology, concurring with Canguilhem's identification of Claude Bernard as "the Newton of the living organism" on the basis of Bernard's elaboration of the "biological concept of the *milieu intérieur*, which at last permitted physiology to be a deterministic science, for the same reason that physics is, without yielding to the fascination of the [mechanical] model which physics offered to it." G. Canguilhem, *Études d'histoire et de philosophie des sciences* (2e éd., Paris, 1970), p. 149. We have already called attention to the relationship between Magendie's theoretical views and Bernard's concept of the *milieu intérieur;* thus we may say that Magendie stood in relation to Bernard, both conceptually and methodologically, as Galileo did to Newton. In relation to his immediate predecessors Magendie's position is equally Galilean, as the second part of this study has attempted to show; also, cf. C. Lichtenthaeler, *Les dates de la Renaissance médicale: Fin de la tradition hippocratique et galénique*, Gesnerus 9 (1952): 8–30. Finally, we may note Magendie's relation to his contemporaries: just as Galileo's mechanics was criticized from the point of view of scholastic

physics, so too was Magendie's physiology attacked by proponents of the system of vital properties. In 1820, for example, Pierre-Adolphe Piorry (1794–1879) attempted a detailed refutation of the theses of Magendie's 1809 paper as they had been summarized in his *Précis*. See F. Magendie, *Elementary Summary*, 1: 12–16; and P.-A. Piorry, *Propriétés*, Dictionaire [*sic*] des sciences médicales (60 v., Paris, 1812–1822), 45: 443–66.

229. We should mention, however, that there were important differences between these two books from the point of view of their internal logic. In a study being prepared for publication (reference 174), I attempt to show (among other things) that the logic of Lavoisier's work was the same as that of Bichat's.

230. C. Bernard, *Éloge de Magendie*, p. 19.

231. F. Magendie, *Some general ideas*, and *Elementary Summary*, 1: ix.

232. G. Canguilhem, *Études*, p. 242.

233. G. Canguilhem, *La connaissance de la vie* (2e éd., Paris, 1971), p. 21.

234. In advancing this conclusion we must bear in mind another of Canguilhem's observations: "Tant que les savants ont conçu les fonctions des organes dans un organisme à l'image des fonctions de l'organisme lui-même dans le milieu extérieur, il était naturel qu'ils empruntassent les concepts de base, les idées directrices de l'explication et de l'expérimentation biologiques à l'expérience pragmatique du vivant humain, puisque c'est un vivant humain qui se trouve être en même temps, et d'ailleurs au titre de vivant, le savant curieux de la solution théorique des problèmes posés par la vie du fait même de son exercice." Ibid., p. 22. We have seen this process of borrowing from human experience illustrated in the work of Bichat and other physiologists of sensibility and contractility. In the case of Magendie, however, the organism in its *milieu extérieur* was not man but the Cuvierian animal; thus the directive idea of Magendie's experimentation was biological rather than anthropomorphic. At the explanatory level, however, Magendie was unable to resolve the conflict between mechanism and vitalism, a resolution which required Bernard's concept of the *milieu intérieur*.

235. C. Bernard, *Éloge de Magendie*, pp. 3–12. We cannot endorse Schiller's statement that Bernard's "historical references . . . take a particular value in view of the place he occupies in the development of modern physiology." J. Schiller, *Physiology's struggle*, p. 72. On the contrary, Bernard's involvement in the scientific controversies of his day makes his historical interpretations extremely suspect. As the following quotation indicates, his approach to history was essentially polemical: "In the history of science it is not enough to recount what everyone may have said, blemished by the errors of each period. It is necessary to characterize each idea, then to criticize it and even to reject things if they are bad, for historical science consists not only in accumulating, but in choosing the useful materials and making them bear fruit." C. Bernard, *The Cahier Rouge of Claude Bernard*, trans. H. H. Hoff, L. Guillemin, and R. Guillemin, in *Claude Bernard and Experimental Medicine*, p. 50 (separately paginated).

236. Cf. M. Foucault, *The Order of Things*, chapters 7 and 8.

237. E.g., M. Foucault, *The Archaeology of Knowledge*, trans. A. Sheridan Smith (New York, 1972); D. Lecourt, *Marxism and Epistemology: Bachelard, Canguilhem and Foucault* (London, 1975); and Louis Althusser and Etienne Balibar, *Reading Capital* (New York, 1970).

238. MS. of twenty-nine pages in the Bibliothèque de la Faculté de Médecine de Paris. The French text of these two lectures was published, in a somewhat abbreviated and corrupted form, by A. Arène in 1911; see M.-F.-X. Bichat, *Discours sur l'étude de phisiologie* [*sic*], ed. A. Arène, Arch. d'anth. crim. 26 (1911): 161–72. The present translation, which restores the passages omitted by Arène, was made from a photocopy of the manuscript obtained for me by Mlle Louise Lafontaine, whose assistance is gratefully acknowledged, and it is published here with the permission of the Bibliothèque de la Faculté de Médecine.

239. Bichat's phrase, which we have rendered throughout as "observational physiology" was "physiologie d'observation"; similarly we have translated "physiologie de raisonnement" as "rational physiology."

240. Cf. Ménuret's treatment of Hippocrates, "le premier et le meilleur de tous les médecins *observateurs*," in J.-J. Ménuret de Chambuad, *Observateur*, p. 291A-B; *Observation*, pp. 296B–297A, 306B–307A; and *Oeconomie animale*, p. 421A-B.

241. Cf. Vicq-d'Azyr's statement that "il ne faut pas considérer l'homme seul; on doit le

rapprocher des autres animaux: ainsi rassemblés, ils forment un tableau imposant par son étendue, et piquant par sa variété,'' and his 1792 table of the functions as manifested in the different classes of animals. F. Vicq-d'Azyr, *Oeuvres recueillies,* 4: 20, 233–37.

242. An illegible word.

243. Cf. J.-J. Ménuret de Chambaud, *Observation,* p. 297B: ''La prétendue découverte de la circulation éblouit tous esprits, augmenta le délire et la fureur des hypothèses, et jeta dans l'esprit des médecins le goût stérile des expériences toujours infructueuses.''

244. See A von Haller, *Mémoires sur la nature sensible et irritable des parties du corps animal* (4 v., Lausanne, 1756–60). Haller's experiments (*Expériences sur la dure-mère et son insensibilité,* ibid., 1; 151–57) and those of his collaborators (ibid., 2: passim) indicated that the dura mater has no sensibility. Haller summarized these findings in his famous *Dissertation sur les parties irritables et sensibles des animaux* (ibid., 1; 26–28; English translation cited in reference 52, above). Other experimenters, however, such as M. A. Caldini, reported finding that the dura mater exhibits sensibility in some circumstances (*Lettre de Marc Antoine Caldini,* ibid., 3: 47–51 and 60–63). Haller attempted to reproduce Caldini's experiments, but could not obtain a similar result (*Expériences nouvelles sur différens animaux vivans,* ibid., 4: 14–18; cf. *Réponse générale aux objections qu'on a faites contre l'insensibilité de plusieurs parties du corps animé,* ibid., 4: 27 ff., and the English *Dissertation,* pp. 46–49). In a paper of 1799 Bichat again referred to ''les résultats très-variés et souvent opposés des expériences faites sur la dure-mère, le périoste, etc. par Haller, Lecat, Caldini, Lamure, etc.'' M.-F.-X. Bichat, *Dissertation sur les membranes, et sur leurs rapports généraux d'organisation,* Mém. de la Soc. méd. d'émulation 2 (1799): 382. For Bichat's explanation of these contradictory results, see our discussion, above.

245. See L. Spallanzani, *Fisica animale e vegetabile, esposta in dissertazione* (Venezia, 1782); and *Expériences de M. Spallanzani sur la digestion de l'homme et de différentes espèces d'animaux,* trans. J. Senebier (Genève, 1783), the latter being a translation into French of the portions of the former work that deal with digestion. Spallanzani's experiments showed that digestion is not a process of fermentation, putrefaction or trituration, as had previously been supposed, but a dissolution effected by the gastric juices. His most striking experiments consisted in the reproduction of the digestive process *in vitro,* using gastric juices obtained from regurgitated sponges.

246. Bichat described his experiments on the gall bladder at several places in his *Traité des membranes.* In numerous experiments comparing the condition of the viscera during the digestive process and during a period of starvation, Bichat found that the gall bladder contains about half as much bile during digestion as it does when the animal is fasting. See M.-F.-X. Bichat, *Traité des membranes,* pp. 20–21, 37–39, and 39n–42n.

247. Bichat's experiments on respiration and asphyxiation took as their starting-point the researches of Edmund Goodwyn, whose 1789 book on *The Connexion of Life with Respiration* (see reference 41, above) was translated into French by J. N. Hallé as ''un modèle de logique expérimentale, c.à.d., de l'art difficile et rare de bien raisonner d'après l'expérience.'' Translator's note in E. Goodwyn, *La connexion de la vie avec la respiration,* pp. 438–39. See M.-F.-X. Bichat, *Recherches physiologiques,* pp. 239–97.

248. Bichat injected various fluids into the body cavities of animals and found that only certain substances were absorbed from these cavities by the lymphatics. See M.-F.-X. Bichat, *Traité des membranes,* pp. 98–102.

249. We have not been able to find examples of experimentation on this subject in Bichat's works.

250. An illegible word, possibly a name. The first experiments on this subject were carried out in 1735 by an English surgeon, John Belchier (1706–85), who noticed that the bones of a pig that fed on madder had become reddened and attempted to produce the same phenomenon in roosters. See J. Belchier, *An account of the bones of animals being changed to a red colour by aliment only,* Phil. Trans. 39 (1734–36): 287–88, and *A further account of the bones of animals being made red by aliment only,* Phil. Trans. 39 (1734–36): 299–300. When news of these experiments was sent to France in 1737, Henri-Louis Duhamel du Monceau (1700–82) undertook a much more elaborate series of experiments upon chickens, pigeons, and turkeys to confirm and extend Belchier's findings. See H.-L. Duhamel du Monceau, *Observations and experiments with*

madder-root, which has the faculty of tinging the bones of living animals of a red colour, Phil. Trans. 41 (1739–41): 390–406. In six additional memoirs on this subject Duhamel was able to show that the growth of bones occurs at their surfaces, by the production of successive layers of new material, rather than throughout the bone by a process of "intussusception" as had previously been thought. See L. Plantefol, *Duhamel du Monceau*, Dix-huit. siècle 1 (1969): 131–33. Experiments such as these served in the late eighteenth and early nineteenth centuries as proof that the bones, the most solid parts of the body (and *a fortiori* the other parts of the body as well) undergo a continual process of composition and decomposition.

251. On the basis of numerous post mortem examinations of his patients and experiments upon dogs, Joseph Lieutand (1703–80) asserted that the size of the spleen varies inversely with the fullness of the stomach. See J. Lieutand, *Relation d'une maladie rare de l'estomac avec quelques observations concernant le méchanisme du vomissement et l'usage de la rate*, Mém. de l'Acad. roy. des sci. (1752): 231–32, and *Anatomie historique et pratique*, éd. Portal (nouv. éd., 2 v., Paris, 1776–77), 2: 243–51. Bichat found, however, that although the size of the spleen may vary, it does not do so in any fixed relationship with the fullness or emptiness of the stomach. He first repeated Lieutaud's experiments by opening a series of dogs whose stomachs were in various states of fullness and comparing their spleens as to size, weight, and appearance. But since these dogs were themselves of different ages and sizes he suspected that he lacked a valid basis of comparison. So he performed the same series of experiments using guinea pigs that were of approximately the same size and condition and found no correlation such as Lieutaud had maintained. See M.-F.-X. Bichat, *Traité des membranes*, pp. 50–53; cf. *Anatomie descriptive*, 5: 55–60.

252. Bichat described this experiment as follows: "I inflated the peritoneal cavity of several guinea pigs with carbonic acid gas [CO_2], hydrogen, oxygen and atmospheric air, in order to see if I could obtain through a serous membrane what I had not accomplished in a mucous membrane [namely, the passage of the gas through the membrane and into the bloodstream]. At the end of these experiments I found no difference in the color of the blood in the abdominal system; it was the same as that in a normal guinea pig which I always killed for comparison." M.-F.-X. Bichat, *Traité des membranes*, p. 72.

253. See reference 252 above, and M.-F.-X. Bichat, *Traité des membranes*, pp. 18–20, where Bichat stated that guinea pigs easily survive artificial emphysema produced by oxygen or carbonic acid gas and that the swelling finally dissipates, little by little.

254. Reading *physiologie* for *anatomie*.

255. Cf. Bichat's reiteration of this point in his *Traité des membranes*, pp. 147–48, and his later study *De l'influence nerveuse dans les sympathies*, J. de méd., chir., pharm. (1801): 472–83.

256. Reading *ainsi* for *aussi*.

257. An illegible word.

258. Conjectured for an illegible word, following Arène.

259. Reading *pas* for *que;* cf. M.-F.-X. Bichat, *Recherches physiologiques*, pp. 92–93.

260. Cf. M.-F.-X. Bichat, *Anatomie générale*, 1: xxxvii; and F. Magendie and R. Delille, *Mémoire sur les organes de l'absorption*, p. 32.

261. Reading *muqeuses* for *sereuses;* cf. M.-F.-X. Bichat, *Traité des membranes*, pp. 74–75, which the rest of this paragraph recapitulates to some extent.

262. An illegible word.

263. The theory of the chemist Antoine Laurent Lavoisier (1743–94) that the moisture of the breath is formed by a chemical union of oxygen from inhaled air with hydrogen from the blood was first propounded in 1785. See A. L. Lavoisier, *Mémoire sur les altérations qui arrivent à l'air dans plusieurs circonstances où se trouve les hommes réunis en société* [1785], Mém. de la Soc. roy de méd. 5 (1782–83): 569–82; reprinted with Lavoisier's revisions in *Oeuvres de Lavoisier*, ed. J. B. Dumas and E. Grimaux (6 v., Paris, 1864–1893), 2: 676–87. Bichat, on the other hand, held that this moisture arose from the dissolution of the mucous exhalations of the lungs and bronchia in the inspired air. He distinguished "exhalations" of fluids from "secretions" by the absence, in the first case, of a specialized gland to produce the fluid. See M.-F.-X. Bichat, *Traité des membranes*, p. 246.

264. Cf. reference 241, above.

265. Although Cabanis's *Rapports du physique et du morale de l'homme* were not published until the year X (1802), the first six memoirs of the twelve contained in this work were read to the *deuxième classe* of the *Institut de France* in the years IV and V, and were printed in *Mémoires de l'Institut national des sciences et arts. Sciences morales et politiques, an* VI [1797–98], *tome* I; and *an* VII [1798–99], *tome* II. Of particular relevance to Bichat's discussion are the second and third memoirs, on the *Histoire physiologique des sensations,* P.-J.-G. Cabanis, *Oeuvres philosophiques,* 1: 164–234.

266. See J. Locke, *An Essay Concerning the Humane Understanding* (London, 1690); and É. B. de Condillac, *Oeuvres philosophiques,* esp. *Essai sur l'origine des connoissances humaines* [1746], 1: 1–118, and *Traité des sensations* [1754], 1: 219–319.

267. Reading *tête* for *coeur;* cf. M.-F.-X. Bichat, *Recherches physiologiques,* pp. 67–68.

268. The "life of relation" was another term used by Bichat for the "exterior life" or "animal life"; cf. M.-F.-X. Bichat, *Mémoire sur les rapports qui existent entre les organes à forme symétrique, et ceux à forme irregulière,* Mém. de la Soc. méd. d'émulation 2 (1799): 477–87.

269. Cf. J.-J. Ménuret de Chambaud, *Observateur,* pp. 287B–288A.

270. An illegible word, probably a name, read by Arène as "Tycho."

271. See G. A. Borelli, *De motu animalium. Opus posthumum* (Romae, 1680–81).

272. Cf. M.-F.-X. Bichat, *Recherches physiologiques,* pp. 93–97.

273. See H. Boerhaave, *Institutiones medicas* (Lugdini, 1708), sect. *Humorum morbi;* and *Aphorismi de cognoscendis et curandis morbis* (Lugdini, 1709), aph. 370–401; cf. J.-J. Ménuret de Chambaud, *Oeconomie animale,* p. 423A.

274. See J. Jurin, *De motu aquarum fluentium,* Phil. Trans. 30 (1717–19), problemata III–VI; J. Keill, *An Account of Animal Secretion, The Quantity of Blood in the Humane Body, and Muscular Motion* (London, 1708), pp. 136 ff., *Concerning the velocity of the blood;* and F. B. de Sauvages de la Croix, *Recherches sur les lois du mouvement du sang dans les vaissaux,* Hist. de l'Acad. roy. des sci. et belles let. de Berlin 11 (1755): 34–55, cf. R. K. French, *Sauvages, Whytt and the motion of the heart: Aspects of eighteenth century animism,* Clio Med. 7 (1972): 35–54. Jurin criticized the portion of Keill's book dealing with the force of the heart in another paper on this subject (J. Jurin, *De potentia cordis dissertatio,* Phil. Trans. 30 [1717–19]: 863–72 and 929–38), to which Keill responded from his deathbed (J. Keill, *De viribus cordis epistola,* Phil. Trans. 30 [1717–19]: 995–1000). These papers, together with Jurin's final word on the matter (J. Jurin, *Epistola . . . qua doctrinam suam De Potentia Cordis contra nuperas Objectiones Viri Clariss. D. Jacobi Keillii, M.D. . . . defendit,* Phil. Trans. 30 (1717–19): 1039–50), were included in the expanded fourth edition of Keill's book, published as: J. Keill, *Essays on Several Parts of the Animal Economy: to Which Is Added a Dissertation Concerning the Force of the Heart by James Jurin, with Dr. Keill's Answer and Dr. Jurin's Reply* (London, 1738). The controversy was typical of the disputes over the force of the heart to which Bichat alluded in his discussion of mechanics, above.

275. Bichat referred here not to Marc-Antoine Petit (1766–1811), the surgeon with whom he studied in Lyons, but to François-Parfour du Petit (1664–1741). The latter regarded the nerves as tubes through which fluid "nervous spirits" were carried. See F.-P. du Petit, *Mémoire dans lequel il est démontré que les nerfs intercostaux fournissent des rameaux qui portent les esprits dans les yeux,* Mém. de l'Acad. roy. des sci. (1727): 1–19, in which he observed that the sectioning of the sympathetic nerve in an animal's neck caused the pupil of the eye to become constricted.

276. See A. L. Lavoisier, *Expériences sur la respiration des animaux et sur les changements qui arrivent à l'air en passant par leur poumon,* Mém. de l'Acad. roy. des sci. (1777): 185–94, reprinted in *Oeuvres de Lavoisier,* 2: 174–83; A. L. Lavoisier and P. S. Laplace, *Mémoire sur la chaleur,* Mém. de l'Acad. roy. des sci. (1780): 355–408, reprinted in *Oeuvres de Lavoisier,* 2: 283–333; and reference 263 above.

277. For the results of Lavoisier's collaboration with Armand Seguin (1765–1835), see A. L. Lavoisier and A. Seguin, *Premier mémoir sur la respiration des animaux,* Mém. de l'Acad. roy. des sci. (1789): 566–84, and *Premier mémoire sur la transpiration des animaux,* Mém. de l'Acad. roy. des sci. (1790): 601–12; reprinted in *Oeuvres de Lavoisier,* 2: 688–703 and 704–14.

278. For a discussion of the prodigious chemical work of Antoine-François Fourcroy (1755–1809) on such topics as the medicinal effects of oxygen and the analysis of animal substances—

particularly calculi, urine, and bones—see W. A. Smeaton, *Fourcroy, Chemist and Revolutionary* (Cambridge, England, 1962), chapter 9: *Animal and Medicinal Chemistry,* pp. 136–62; and the bibliography of Fourcroy's journal articles to 1798, ibid., pp. 237–41.

279. Louis Jurine (1751–1819) was well known at this time for his prize-winning essay on eudiometry, which included chemical analyses of the changes which air undergoes in respiration, both by healthy and sick individuals, an attempt to discover whether any air passes out of the body through the skin, a study of the ambient air in certain morbid states, and finally researches on the composition of intestinal gases. See L. Jurine, *Mémoire sur la question suivante proposé par la Société royale de médecine: Déterminer quels avantages la médecine peut retirer des découvertes modernes sur l'art de connaitre la pureté de l'air par les différens eudiomètres,* Mém. de la Soc. roy. de méd. 10 (1798): 19 ff.

280. An illegible word.

281. Conjectured for an illegible word, following Arène.

282. See A.-F. Fourcroy, *Mémoire sur la nature de la fibre charnue ou musculaire et sur la siège de l'irritabilité,* Mém. de la Soc. roy. de méd. 3 (1782–83): 502–13; and W. A. Smeaton, *Fourcroy,* pp. 139–40.

283. An illegible word. For Jurine's researches on intestinal gases, see reference 279 above.

284. A translation of pp. 76–79 of G. Cuvier, *Histoire de la classe des sciences mathématiques et physiques,* Mém. de l'Inst. nat. des sci. et arts: Sci. math. et phys. 7 (1806): 1–79, with title supplied by myself.

285. See reference 129 above.

286. Cf. the following remarks from Magendie's *Précis* of 1816; "We must not abuse the meaning of this term *vital power;* it signifies, and can only signify, the *unknown cause* of the phenomena of life. Just as attraction, say physiologists, presides over the changes of condition in inert bodies, [so too] does the vital power govern the modifications of organised bodies; but they fall into a strange error, for the vital force cannot be compared to attraction; the laws of the latter are perfectly known, those of the vital power are perfectly unknown. Physiology is, with respect to it, at this moment, exactly at the point at which the physical sciences were before the time of Newton: waiting for some genius of the first order, to discover the laws of the vital power, as Newton discovered those of attraction. The glory of this mathematician does not consist in having discovered attraction, as some believe, for this cause was already known; but in having said, that *attraction acts in the direct ratio of the mass, and the inverse ratio of the square of the distance.*" F. Magendie, *Elementary Summary,* 1: 11. According to Schiller, "For all [Magendie's] contemporaries, Newton discovered the law of universal gravitation. For him alone, as he affirmed later [1816], Newton discovered that bodies attract each other in the direct ratio of their masses and the inverse ratio of the square of the distance." J. Schiller, *Claude Bernard,* p. 45. We see, however, that Cuvier's position on this matter in 1806 (with its emphasis upon determining "the measure and laws by which [gravitational] attractions act" and on "the agreement between rigorous calculation and precise observations") was in all important respects the same as that taken by Magendie a decade later.

287. In his 1807 lectures Cuvier also gave prominence to experimentation as a means of investigating organic phenomena. As Coleman reports, "he argued that there can be only two kinds of explanations in the sciences, the physical and the nonphysical. When our ideal explanation (the physical) fails, we should turn not to speculation but to experimentation. To propose a vital force is 'ridiculous, meaningless', and defeatist. One must follow the example of physics and, just as Newton analyzed the problem of attraction into its individual instances, so must the physiologist remove the complexities from his problems. Cuvier developed this argument by contrasting the ideas and work of Haller and of P. J. Barthez.... Haller's memoir of 1756 had shown how so-called vital forces could be reduced to the experimentally meaningful concepts of irritability and sensibility. Barthez, Cuvier felt, had followed a reactionary course and refused to admit his ignorance.... The physiologist gained nothing from vague hypotheses, since chemistry, anatomy, and experimentation alone could lead to positive and therefore useful results." W. Coleman, *Georges Cuvier,* pp. 36–37.

288. Cf. the comparisons made between physiology and the physical sciences by Bichat and by Cuvier in the texts translated above.

289. Reading *plus* for *peu.*

290. Reading *peu exacts* for *plus exacts*.

291. See the *Synoptic Table* of Professor Chaussier [Magendie's note]. Chaussier's complete definition of sensibility was as follows: "Sensibility: Faculty of feeling, that is to say, of experiencing by the contact of a foreign body a more or less profound impression which changes the *natural and usual rhythm* of vibratility or of motility proper to the parts, which impresses upon them a more or less remarkable order of movement which tends to isolate them, to move them away from or to move them closer to the object which touches them." F. Chaussier, *Table synoptique . . . de la force vitale*.

292. Idem [Magendie's note]. The following was Chaussier's full definition of motility: "Motility: Faculty of movement—a property of organic solids—which consists in a continual tendency toward contraction or tightening or shortening, which produces and maintains in all the fibres, all the vessels and all the tissues, a movement which determines the progression of the fluids." Ibid.

293. For a description of these experiments see reference 250, above.

294. Another phenomenon that is observed in all organized bodies is the production of heat—a production that gives them, in the most usual cases, a temperature independent of that of their surrounding bodies. The majority of the physiologists consider the heat proper to living bodies as a secondary phenomenon of the nutritive movement. Professor Chaussier has made it one of the properties that manifest the vital force, but since the nature of caloric is still uncertain I believe it would be most wise to wait until the opinion of the physicists on the nature of caloric becomes entirely fixed before seeking to explain the production of vital heat in a rigorous manner.

In the meantime we can easily be content with the received explanation, which furthermore accords quite well with the admitted theory concerning the cause of heat [Magendie's note]. Chaussier offered the following definition of caloricity in his *Synoptic Table:* "Caloricity: Faculty of releasing or of developing a certain quantity of caloric and of resisting atmospheric cold by this means, of maintaining and conserving in all parts a nearly-equal temperature at all times, and of contributing to the fluidity of the juices and to the vaporization of some of them." F. Chaussier, *Table synoptique . . . de la force vitale*. The uncertainty concerning the nature of heat, to which Magendie referred, arose from the coexistence, at the time, of two theories of heat, one of which regarded it as an imponderable fluid, while the other treated it as a product of a molecular motion. See A. L. Lavoisier and P. S. Laplace, *Mémoire sur la chaleur*. For Bichat's rejection of "caloricity" see M.-F.-X. Bichat, *Recherches physiologiques,* p. 131.

295. It will presently be seen that there are some parts of living bodies that do not seem to have any action at all and that are limited to the nutritive movement: the bones, the cartilage, the exteriors of crustaceans, the solid parts of zoophytes, etc. [Magendie's note].

296. Cf. Bichat's statement that "The perfection of animals, if I may speak thus, is in proportion to the dose of this [animal] sensibility which they have received." M.-F.-X. Bichat, *Recherches physiologiques,* p. 100.

297. Cf. Bichat's remark on the need for seeking causes in his *Discourse*.

298. Cf. Georges L. Duvernoy's application of this principle to medicine in 1799: ". . . since life is manifested by differing phenomena among differently organized beings in the state of health, it should develop varied phenomena among these same beings in the diseased state. Thus, the same causes will differently modify the different organized bodies upon which they simultaneously act. These modifications will be the more similar as the organization of the beings which experience them is more analogous." G. L. Duvernoy, *Réflexions sur les Corps organisés et les sciences dont ils sont l'objet,* Mag. encyclopédique 5[3] (1799): 459–60. Duvernoy (1777–1855) was an enthusiastic student of Cuvier's at this time (ibid., p. 174) and subsequently edited the last three volumes of the latter's *Leçons d'anatomie comparée* for publication.

299. Magendie persisted in this opinion throughout his career. In 1839, for example, he told his students, "Anatomy, and above all, microscopical anatomy, has in recent times made admirable researches into the structure and the molecular disposition of the nervous system; and we shall attempt to connect these discoveries to the mechanism of the nervous functions." F. Magendie, *Les fonctions et les maladies,* 1: 18. Later in the same lecture series, however, he warned his students against drawing conclusions too hastily from "the microscopical anatomy of the nervous system," reminding them that it was "a completely new science." Ibid., 2: 6–7.

300. Cf. Bichat's rejection of these special forces in M.-F.-X. Bichat, *Recherches physiologiques,* p. 131.

301. Reading *de* for *ou*.

302. See reference 268, above.

303. See, for example, M.-F.-X. Bichat, *Mémoire sur les rapports,* p. 478, and *Recherches physiologiques,* p. 5.

304. Ibid.

305. Under the term, brain, I include the spinal cord [Magendie's note].

306. Reading *au* for *du*.

307. Cf. Bichat's attack on theories of "nervous atmospheres," "fluids," etc., in M.-F.-X. Bichat, *Anatomie générale,* 1: 173–74.

308. *Synoptic Table* [Magendie's note]. Magendie was probably referring here to Chaussier's *Table synoptique des sensations* (Paris, s.d.), which we have unfortunately not been able to consult.

309. "M. Dupuytren, in the general anatomy course that he gave this year at the Hôtel-Dieu, benefited greatly from this manner of regarding animal sensibility and contractility. I also employed it with success in the physiology course that I gave this year at the College of Medical Students" [Magendie's note]. Guillaume Dupuytren (1777–1835) was named chirurgien-adjoint at the Hôtel Dieu in 1808. A protégé of Chaussier at the time, he undertook a series of physiological experiments as a result of the older man's encouragement. Shortly afterward, however, he devoted himself primarily to surgery, becoming by 1815 the most prominent surgeon in France and maintaining that position until his death. See L. Delhoume, *Dupuytren* (3e éd., Paris, 1935), pp. 35, 52, and passim; and H. Mondor, *Dupuytren* (2e éd., Paris, 1945), p. 28 and passim. For information on the College of Medical Students, a private institution in Paris offering a complete education in medicine with four years of courses paralleling those at the École de Médecine, see E. Wickesheimer, *Une institution oubliée: le Collège des Étudians en Médecine de la rue Saint-Victor,* La France méd. 54 (1907): 117–19.

Nature and Nurture: The Interplay of Biology and Politics in the Work of Francis Galton

Ruth Schwartz Cowan

In the nineteenth century the study of heredity, and most especially the study of human heredity, was fraught with political overtones, as indeed it is still today. Francis Galton (1822–1911) was one of the founders of anthropometry and population genetics, two of the sciences that now converge on the study of human heredity. He was also one of the founders of the eugenics movement, and this coincidence was not accidental. Galton's committment to the ideal of a eugenic society is the single most important clue to understanding the direction and the import of the work that he did in genetics, statistics, psychology, and anthropology. His plan for a eugenic society was based on his belief that heredity was omnicompetent—to use more familiar terminology—that nature was more important than nurture in determining the character of the human race. This belief was already fully formed in 1864 when Galton began to study heredity (he was then forty-two years old) and in subsequent years it was the light that guided him down the often torturous paths of scientific discovery.[1]

Galton's political and social ideas imposed themselves upon his scientific work in various ways, one of the most crucial of which was the creation of a kind of differential skepticism. He was willing to accept some scientific ideas and insisted upon rejecting others, when the scientific evidence that was available was inconclusive at best and insubstantial at worst. This differential skepticism was most clearly displayed in an article that Galton wrote for *Macmillan's Magazine,* in 1865, reporting the results of his first empirical study of human heredity.[2] A close analysis of this article provides a useful insight into the differentially skeptical mind at work, and it also helps to

---

Ruth Schwartz Cowan, State University of New York at Stony Brook.

clarify some of the political and social issues that were at stake in the nineteenth-century debate about heredity.

The article opens, in its very first paragraph, with a clear statement of the eugenic principle: "The power of man over animal life, in producing whatever varieties of form he pleases is enormously great. It would seem as though the physical structure of future generations was almost as plastic as clay, under the control of the breeder's will. It is my desire to show more pointedly than—so far as I am aware—has been attempted before, *that mental qualities are equally under control* [italics added]."[3] Stated this way the idea seems simple but its ramifications are complex and enormous in number. Galton hoped that his ideas about mental heredity would produce a political and religious reformation of society. That, he realized, would be no easy task and in order to accomplish it he had to prove that mental qualities were in fact inherited, and that inheritance was the only major determinant of mental ability.

He commenced that proof by presenting two analogies: between physical and mental heredity, and between heredity in man and heredity in other animals. He argued that heredity operates just as forcibly in man as it does in beasts, since two generations of humans are as likely to resemble each other as two generations of horses, dogs, or cats. Thus, if we had proof of the inheritance of mental ability in animals we would have grounds for believing that such abilities can also be inherited by men.

Unfortunately, this proof did not exist, since animals had never been bred for intelligence. This was an obstacle to Galton's argument, but one which did not deter him for very long; he simply asserted that the mental resemblance between animals of the same species was very strong and that therefore it was probably due to hereditary influences—and that the same could be said for human species. Galton's argument was somewhat circular, but he did not seem to realize that; neither did he recognize the possibility that some influence other than heredity might be at work.

"Resemblance frequently fails where we might have expected it to hold"; Galton admitted, "but we may fairly ascribe the failure to the influence of conditions that we do not yet comprehend" (p. 158). After all, resemblance does not invariably hold with regard to the physical features of domestic animals, but breeders can still create new strains when they wish to. "They [the breeders] know, with accurate prevision, when particular types of animals are mated together, what will be the character of the offspring." And, said Galton, "I maintain by analogy that his prevision could be equally attained in respect to the mental qualities, though I cannot prove it" (p. 158).

Up to this point Galton's argument was little more than a logical construct, but then he proceeded to concrete evidence. "I can show," he said, "that talent and peculiarities of character are found in the children when they have existed in either of the parents, to an extent beyond all question greater than in the children of ordinary persons" (p. 158). His evidence was derived from statistical analyses of biographical dictionaries.

He had determined the number of famous men listed in one such dictionary (Phillips, *The Million of Facts*) and then he had calculated the number of familial relationships among them. Out of 605 individuals, 102 were relatives of someone else on the list; the frequency of talented men who were related to each other was, in this case, 1 in 6. Although Galton realized that some of the people on his list did not deserve the label "talented" (for example, four male members of the House of Orange), he argued that other names could have been substituted if those had been removed (two Hallams, for instance) and that "the overwhelming force of a statistical fact like this renders counter-arguments of no substantial effect" (p. 160).

The analysis continued in a similar vein. From another biographical list Galton culled 1,141 names; out of these 103 were related, a frequency of 1 in 11. A third list (of "living notables") yielded a frequency of 1 in 3 ½; a fourth (of painters) produced the ratio 1 in 6, and a fifth (musicians) produced 1 in 10.

At this point in the presentation of his evidence Galton stopped to admit that, "when a parent has achieved great eminence, his son will be placed in a more favourable position for advancement, than if he had been the son of an ordinary person" (p. 161). Although this is true, Galton maintained, of those who enter political and military careers, it is not true of those who enter the fields of science and literature. These fields are "open"—by which he meant that only a good education can give one man advantage over another of equal ability. Thus, if the same rough ratio were found to exist for literary and scientific men the objection of "family influence" could be eliminated. Sure enough, taking 300 names of scientists and writers from Phillips's list of talented men, Galton found the ratio of relatives among them to be 1 in 12. Similarly, among lord chancellors—the law being, according to Galton, "by far the most open to fair competition of all the professions" (p. 161)—13 out of 39 had eminent kinsmen, a ratio of 1 in 3.

With a few more statistics and one summarizing sentence—"Everywhere is the enormous power of hereditary influence forced on our attention" (p. 163)—Galton rested his case. Rarely in the history of science has such an important generalization been made on the basis of so little concrete evidence, so badly put, and so naively conceived. Nearly every paragraph of this opening section of Galton's article contains something that could have been easily disputed in his time. The most fundamental weakness in his argument lay in the very empirical materials upon which he had founded it. He had set out to prove "that talent and peculiarities of character are found in the children, when they have existed in either of the parents, to an extent beyond all question greater than in the children of ordinary persons" (158), but his statistics revealed *nothing* about the frequency of talented children born to ordinary persons. They did not even reveal much about the *children* of talented parents, because, more often than not, the relationship between the men on his lists had been that of brothers, cousins, uncles, nephews, and grandparents. Worse yet, none of Galton's statistics give him valid grounds for eliminating the environmental conditions that might have produced the results he found. [4]

Francis Galton was not a stupid man, nor a man untrained in mathematics, nor a man inexperienced in affairs of the world. He had studied mathematics with a private tutor when a boy and had read mathematics at Cambridge. In 1865 he was secretary of the British Association, had been a secretary of the Royal Geographic Society, and was on the management committee of Kew Observatory. How could a reasonably intelligent man, with a reasonable grasp of mathematics and a reasonable amount of experience of the world have made judgments as naïve as the ones that appear in "Hereditary Talent and Character?"

If, in 1865, it was commonly accepted that mental ability is the product of hereditary influences, or if it was commonly held that men could be bred for their mental capacity just as animals could be bred for physical ability, Galton's apparent naïveté would make more sense. For if Galton was merely reaffirming what had already been established as fact, he would have had no need to worry over the loopholes in his argument. Commonly recognized truths do not need to be reestablished each time that they are discussed.

But "mental heredity" was not a commonly recognized truth in the 1860s; the dominant ideological current at that time, both in England and in the United States, was environmentalism, the conviction that environmental conditions were the prime determinants of mental ability. [5] When Galton elaborated "Hereditary Talent and Character" into a book, *Hereditary Genius* (published in 1869), several reviewers of the book commented on the novelty of his argument. One of them wrote, for example:

Had not [the] process of accustoming Public Opinion to a sharp pace and difficult leaps been going on for some time, it is to be believed that Mr. Galton's book would have produced considerably more dismay and called forth more virtuous indignation than under present training has actually greeted it. We have had to modify our ideas of all things in heaven and earth so fast, that *another shock even to our conceptions of the nature of our own individual minds and faculties,* is not so terrible as it would once have been [italics added]. [6]

Galton's views on mental heredity were unorthodox in two respects; they contradicted traditional theological teachings about the origin of the mind, and they also contradicted more "objective," scientific ideas on the same subject.

Viewed theologically, the notion that a man's mental faculties were bequeathed to him by his ancestors contradicted the notion that a man's mental faculties were bequeathed to him by God. In short, and this did not go unnoticed by Galton's critics, the idea of mental heredity denied the existence of a God-given soul:

There have always been some sacred regions to which the man who could not part with faith in the living God has prided himself that even Materialism could not penetrate. The *Ego,* the individuality, that which constituted the centre of his consciousness, has said, "I came forth from God." "Parents have been instrumental in God's hands in fashioning my physical frame, and even my animal temperament and the quality which my nature has assumed, but God is the father of my spirit." This respectable delusion is now swept away by . . . our author [Galton].[7]

Theological objections aside, Galton's ideas were also disconcerting to some of the "advanced thinkers" of his time because they were not in accord with notions then current in philosophy, ethnology, psychology, or any other field of endeavor that dealt with the problems of the mind. Environmentalism dominated those fields in the 1860s and continued to do so almost until the turn of the century.

The most extreme form of environmentalism had been propounded in the previous century by followers of Locke and Condillac, who maintained that at the time of birth the brain is a *tabula rasa* and that all abilities, qualities, faculties, and ideas possessed by an adult have actually been acquired during the course of his own life and cannot under any circumstances be passed on to his offspring. Among English writers David Hartley (1705–57) was a good example of an extreme environmentalist.[8] For most of the nineteenth century a more moderate environmentalist position dominated; it differed from the extreme position in maintaining that *acquired* mental faculties could be passed from one generation to the next. This was often referred to as "hereditarianism" in order that it might be distinguished from the complete environmentalism of the Lockeans.[9] Some of the moderate environmentalists, Gall and Spurzheim for example, believed that the brain is composed of several innate faculties, anatomically localized and derived by inheritance from the previous generation. These faculties, depending on the level of their development, were thought to make the individual more or less capable of learning, much as the level of development of a muscle makes an individual more or less capable of moving.[10] Other moderate environmentalists denied the phrenologist's notion of localized faculties, but still maintained that the mind has certain innate abilities. Herbert Spencer, for example, believed that these abilities were actually the accumulated experiences of past generations.[11]

During the mid-Victorian years moderate environmentalism of one sort or another was the theoretical foundation that underlay most proposals for political reform. Many American and British reform movements, such as those for temperance, humane treatment of the insane, and rehabilitation of criminals, were premised on assumptions that had been popularized by the phrenologists, Gall and Spurzheim.[12] The temperance movement, for example, adopted the notion that alcohol would cause physical degeneration of the mental faculties. Humane treatment of the insane was advocated on the grounds that an insane man is suffering from nothing more than a physical disease, some sort of deformity of the brain tissue. An ever-present corollary of all these assumptions was the notion that if a man leads a healthy life, develops all his faculties to their fullest, and marries a woman similarly inclined, his children will be greatly improved:

A man of fair average intellect and good constitution marries a woman similarly endowed. He leads a life free at once from excesses and from asceticism, from torpor and from exhaustive over work,—free, above all things from anxiety. Suppose one of his children, born under such favourable circumstances, well nurtured and well educated, repeats the process. The grandchildren will, in all probability, show marks of decided superiority. If, now such conditions are continued, the result in the fourth or fifth generation may be a Shakspeare [sic] a Bacon or a Humboldt.[13]

But moderate environmentalism, the belief in the inheritance of acquired mental characteristics, pervaded much more than just Victorian politics. Popular and professional medical texts were full of advice about how to conceive happier and healthier children, and most of this advice focussed on the idea that the condition of the child was determined by the condition of the parents at the time of conception: ''As few may be aware of the real importance of that critical period in which life is conferred upon a new being, we have thought it right to put our married readers at least upon their guard against unrestrained yielding to many of the baser feelings or ideas, which do creep into the best regulated establishments.''[14]

The subject of hereditary disease was also much discussed during this period, and it was commonly assumed that there were some diseases which, when they occur during the life of a parent invariably become congenital in the children.[15] In addition, some sort of environmentalism characterized almost all nineteenth-century ethnological theories, ranging from the extreme notions of Buckle—that no racial characteristic can be passed by heredity but only by education and training—to the more moderate opinions of such writers as Prichard, Blumenbach, and Broca, who maintained that racial characters, while inherited, originate as adaptive responses to environmental conditions.[16]

Thus, when Galton adopted a complete hereditarian position, when he maintained that inheritance is the *sole* determinant of mental characteristics he set himself apart from the mainstream of British thought in the nineteenth century. When he asserted that men could be bred for physical ability, when he implied, thereby, that only proper breeding could produce a real improvement in the human race, he was not reaffirming an already established truth, but proposing one that was new and somewhat startling. Somewhat later Galton realized that he had been a bit ahead of his time: "Popular feeling was not then ripe to accept even the elementary truths of hereditary talent and character. . . . Still less was it prepared to consider dispassionately any proposals for practical action. So I laid the subject wholly to one side for many years. Now [1908] I see my way better, and an appreciative audience is at last to be had, though it be small."[17] A brief perusal of Galton's writings after 1865 indicates that he did not, by any means, lay the subject to one side, but his recollection is at least correct on the matter of public willingness to accept his new doctrine. As his wife put it, somewhat despondently, in her diary for the year 1869: "Frank's book 'Hereditary Genius' published in November, but not well received."[18]

Thus Galton's methodology was lax, not because the theory of mental heredity was so well established as to need no rigorous proof, but for some other reason. One need not read much farther into "Hereditary Talent and Character" to discover what that reason was.

Following the presentation of his factual evidence, and without any rhetorical transition, Galton turned to some of the practical objections that might be raised against his scheme to breed men from their intellectual ability. First he disposed of the time-honored notion that there was an inverse relation between intelligence and fertility; then he considered various social conventions—celibacy of the clergy, for one—which had in the past mitigated against the breeding of bigger and better human beings.

In a very short time Galton arrived at the point he had wanted to make all along—the perfect society is one that has adopted "race improvement" as the basis for its ethical code—and he began to sketch an evangelical vision of what the customs of such a society might be like. A series of examinations would identify the ten most talented young men and women in the realm. At a public ceremony they could be given awards and told that if they should—for the good of the State—decide to marry one another, they would each be given £5000 as a wedding present, and the State would defray the cost of educating their children.

If a twentieth part of the cost and pains were spent in measures for the improvement of the human race that is spent on the improvement of the breed of horses and cattle, what a galaxy of genius might we not create! We might introduce prophets and high priests of civilization into the world. . . . Men and Women of the present day are, to those we might hope to bring into existence, what the pariah dogs of the streets of an Eastern town are to our own highly-bred varieties (pp. 165–66).

"Pariah dogs," "galaxies of geniuses," "prophets and high priests of civilization"—these are not expressions normally used in sedate scientific treatises. "Hereditary Talent and Character" was clearly not such a treatise. In some respects it was an exercise in political propaganda, in other respects a personal, emotional testament. Galton's attachment to the idea of mental heredity went far beyond what was warranted by the scientific evidence he had adduced. He had convinced himself of the validity of mental heredity, not because he thought it was a solution to a great scientific problem, but because he was fascinated by the social programs that could be built around it.

This predilection became even more pronounced when he turned to a discussion of the inheritance of mental traits other than intelligence—character traits such as honesty and reliability, personality traits such as gregariousness and religiosity. Here his argument was based on ethnological rather than statistical evidence.

Galton began by asserting that there was a physiological connection between physique and personality; people with combative temperaments have faces that are square, coarse, and heavy-jawed, while people who are ascetic have a distinctly different appearance. This truth was commonly accepted, Galton said, as was the notion that a man's physique came to him by inheritance. If there was a physiological connection between physique and personality, then personality must also be inherited.

This principle was clearly illustrated in ethnology, according to Galton, since each human race was characterized by a unique set of physical attributes as well as a unique temperament. "The Mongolians, Jews, Negroes, Gipsies, and American Indians severally propagate their kinds; and each kind differs in character and intellect, as well as in colour and shape from the other four" (p. 320).

For almost a century students of ethnology had believed that racial temperaments were determined by environment. According to Galton this principle was incorrect; he cited the example of the American Indians to prove his point. The members of this race were spread over an enormous geographical area, through every type of climate and topology. They lived in thousands of different communities, with thousands of different social institutions, spoke many different languages and had been dominated by dozens of different conquering powers. Despite all this, many observers agreed that the race of American Indians,

. . . has fundamentally the same character throughout the whole of America. The men, and in a less degree the women, are naturally cold, melancholic, patient, and taciturn. A father, mother, and their children, are said to live together in a hut, like persons assembled by accident, not tied by affection. The youths treat their parents with neglect . . . the mothers have been seen to commit infanticide without the slightest discomposure. . . . They nourish a sullen reserve, and show little sympathy with each other, even in great distress. . . . The nature of the American Indians appears to contain the minimum of affectionate and social qualities compatible with the continuance of their race (p. 321).

Galton mentioned a few other races for whom a similar argument might be made—West African Negroes, Hindus, Arabs, Teutons—but did not elaborate any farther. He concluded that the universality of the Indian temperament proved that mental dispositions must be hereditary and added that this implied that men might be bred for their dispositions as easily as for intelligence. This said, he ended the presentation of his ethnological evidence.

Once again, Galton's factual argument ended almost before it began. If he was aware that the question he had raised—that of the origin of racial characteristics—had been debated for over a century he did not indicate his awareness. The names of Prichard, Blumenbach, Buffon, or Rousseau did not appear in his article, and Galton did not mention the fact that any number of ethnologists had come to an entirely different conclusion about the origin of racial characteristics. He did not even intimate that the question might actually be difficult to answer. He merely asserted that racial characteristics persisted through generations, then concluded that they must be hereditary and proceeded to other matters.

These other matters were: first, the theory of the inheritance of acquired characters; second, the existence of a God-given soul; third, the origin of religious sentiments; and fourth, the Christian doctrine of original sin. This may seem an unusual combination of topics, but Galton, as we shall see, thought that there were definite connections between them.

He began with the doctrine of the inheritance of acquired mental abilities, the doctrine that had been so attractive to the phrenologists and Victorian social reformers. Were this doctrine to be proven true Galton's scheme for controlled human breeding would be useless; an individual would be able to improve upon or destroy whatever qualities his parents had handed down to him. In such a situation the qualities of the parents would be of little account; all that would matter is what an individual made of what he had. This situation would be inimical in Galton's utopian state, a state in which control of breeding is thought to be the only effective way to improve the human race.

Thus it is not surprising that Galton was opposed to the doctrine of the inheritance of acquired characteristics. His argument emphasized human qualities rather than the physiological or morphological qualities that might have been interesting to a biologist. He was not, at least at this point in his life, concerned about the biological aspects of the problem.

"Can we hand anything down to our children, that we have fairly won by our own independent exertions? Will our children be born with more virtuous dispositions, if we ourselves have acquired virtuous habits? Or are we no more than passive transmitters of a nature we have received, and which we have no power to modify'' (pp. 321–22)?

Galton's answer to the first two questions was, emphatically, ''No.'' Equally emphatically his answer to the third, was ''Yes.'' There was no reliably documented example of inherited habits among animals. Those cases that were documented, cases of dogs that were born with the ability to point or other dogs that demonstrated great affection for their masters immediately after birth, could be explained on other grounds. Most probably, he said, pointing and affection for humans were part of the natural disposition of all dogs. Furthermore, there were, according to Galton, endless examples of characteristics which were firmly engrained in one or both parents but which were never passed down to their offspring. The sons of soldiers did not learn to drill any faster than the sons of other men, nor were the sons of sailors noticeably more accustomed to the sea than the sons of landbound men. Thus, Galton concluded, if acquired habits were transmitted from one generation to the next, they were transmitted to such a slight degree as to be hardly noticeable.

If this was the case, if acquired traits could not be transmitted, how could we understand the relationship between one generation and the next?

We shall therefore take an approximately correct view of the origin of our life, if we consider our own embryos to have sprung immediately from those embryos whence our parents were developed, and these from the embryos of *their* parents, and so on forever. We should in this way look on the nature of mankind, and perhaps on that of the whole animated creation, as one continuous system, ever pushing out new branches in all directions, that variously interlace, and that bud into separate lives at every point of interlacement (p. 322).

Of all the things that Galton wrote in ''Hereditary Talent and Character,'' this paragraph is, beyond any doubt, the most remarkable. He ended his argument against the inheritance of acquired characteristics with a rough statement of the principle of the continuity of germ plasm, the principle that we usually associate with the name of August Weismann and with the year 1883.[19] The principle of continuity of germ plasm lies at the foundation of modern biology. It asserts that nothing passes between parent and child except that which is contained in the nucleus of the fertilized egg. Weismann came to his conclusions on biological grounds, but the same cannot be said of Galton. A few years after writing ''Hereditary Talent and Character'' Galton did create a physiological theory of heredity that embodied the principle of continuity of germ plasm (the stirp theory), but this article of 1865 demonstrates that originally that idea was the result of sociopolitical rather than biological imperatives.[20]

The idea of continuity of germ plasm was absolutely essential to Galton's eugenic scheme; without it the scheme would have very little social utility. The notion of choosing a mate because of his or her biological qualities was somewhat repugnant, but that repugnance could be overcome if people could be made to see that that was the only viable way to improve their families and the race. If the continuity of germ plasm were proven false, then there might be other viable ways to achieve the same ends, ways which were quicker and less repugnant. If the continuity of germ plasm were false, then environmental reform should be just as effective as eugenic reform. From Galton's point of view, past history had clearly demonstrated the failure of environmental reform, therefore—if we follow his logic—the continuity of germ plasm had to be a valid biological hypothesis.

Unless we understand that Galton's convictions about germinal continuity have sociopolitical roots it is difficult to understand why he steadfastly ignored the biological implications of the idea. The inheritance or noninheritance of acquired characteristics had been a thorn in the side of biology for almost a century.[21] Hosts of nineteenth-century biologists, Darwin foremost among them, had realized that there was precious little evidence in support of the doctrine, yet they had been unable to dispense with it because without it certain evolutionary phenomena were inexplicable—or only explicable as examples of special creation.[22] Surely if Galton had been aware of the history of this problem he would have expressed either his regrets or his pleasure at having disposed of the troublesome doctrine once and for all. But we hear nothing of it; Galton apparently delivered the death blow to the inheritance of acquired characters without even a twinge of conscience. In 1865 he seemed to have been completely oblivious to the biological consequences of the doctrine he had enunciated in two short sentences. The inheritance of acquired characteristics was merely an obstacle that stood in the way of his proposal for controlled human breeding.

One more obstacle to the efficacy of that utopian scheme remained to be demolished before Galton's argument would be finished, and here the theological implications of the doctrine of mental heredity began to appear. Earlier he had shown, at least to his own satisfaction, that events which occurred during the life of the adult could not have affected the quality of the offspring. Yet there might be one other factor that could have affected the child before its birth—God. He might have implanted something of the divine spirit in the mind or the body of the child. Galton dispensed with this objection as surely and as swiftly as he had dealt with the more secular theories of the environmentalists.

Most persons seem to have a vague idea that a new element, especially fashioned in heaven, and not transmitted by simple descent, is introduced into the body of every newly-born infant. . . . It is impossible that this should be true, unless there exists some property or quality in man that is not transmissible by descent. But the terms *talent* and *character* are exhaustive. They include the whole of man's spiritual nature. . . . Moreover the idea is improbable from *a priori* considerations, because there is no other instance in which creative power operates under our own observation at the present day, except it may be in the freedom in action of our own wills (p. 322).

Earlier Galton had deftly ignored two long-standing scientific disputes; one about the origin of racial characteristics and the other about the inheritance of acquired qualities. Now, in one short paragraph, he dismissed almost 2,000 years of theological argument about the nature of the soul by simply asserting that it does not exist.

Aside from the soul there were two other religious notions that drew Galton's verbal fire: the so-called "religious sentiments" and the concept of original sin. Using the principle of mental heredity as a base, he argued that these notions were nothing more than phenomena produced by the processes of evolution. There were certain character traits that were advantageous for the survival of the human species, given the fact that humans tend to live in social groups. "There must be affection, and it must be of four kinds: sexual, parental, filial, and social. The absolute deficiency of any one of these would be a serious hindrance, if not a bar to the continuance of any race. Those who possessed all of them in the strongest measure, would, speaking generally, have an advantage in the struggle for existence" (p. 323).

Without sexual affection there will be no children; unless parents care for their children the children will die; unless the members of families support one another the families will disintegrate; and unless families band together societies will be destroyed. This was not a remarkable argument, but Galton put an unusual twist into it. He believed that the four "affections" that insure the survival of the species were, when translated into other words, nothing more nor less than the "religious sentiments." "I believe that our religious sentiments spring primarily from these four sources. The institution of celibacy is an open acknowledgment that the theistic and human affections are more or less convertible. . . . *All evidence tends to show that man is directed to the contemplation and love of God by instincts that he shares with the whole animal world"* [italics added] (p. 324).

There, for the moment, Galton let the matter rest. Before taking up the subject of original sin he digressed for a few pages to discuss matters of nontheological import. Having made a devastating antireligious thrust, he swiftly turned to other less controversial topics. First he discussed the ethnology of the North American continent, attempting to prove that the conditions of life on that continent had insured that only men with violent dispositions would be able to survive. Then he turned to the question of whether or not the English had a national disposition. That, he said, was difficult to determine because the race of Englishmen was relatively new, "but eight hundred years or twenty-six generations since the conquest," and because there had been so many infusions of boorish stock into each of the original noble Norman families. "The share that a man retains in the constitution of his remote descendants is inconceivably small. The father transmits, on an average, one half of his nature, the grandfather, one fourth, the great-grandfather, one-eighth; the share decreasing step by step in a geometrical ratio, with great rapidity" (p. 326).

Such was Galton's first statement of the Law of Ancestral Heredity, the law so often attached to his name. The law did not demonstrate his adherence to the concept of blending inheritance; he probably would not have known what "blending inheritance" was if he had been asked. As the law was first expressed in 1865 it served as little more than an alternative rhetorical device; it enabled him to reiterate his point without repeating the same words twice. "The descendants of Normans have no special claim to nobility," was all that Galton meant to say. As is the case with the principle of continuity of germ plasm, he somewhat later discovered that his computation of the amount that each ancestor contributed to inheritance had biological relevance; only then did he bother to worry about whether or not the fractions he had stated were actually precise.[23]

This short peroration on the value of eugenic planning brought Galton almost to the end of "Hereditary Talent and Character," and he turned for one last assault upon theological dogma, this time the concept of original sin. To Galton, the concept of original sin was a social construct which acknowledged the disparity between the evolution of civilization and the evolution of man.

It is a common theme of moralists of many creeds, that a man is born with an imperfect nature. He has lofty aspirations, but there is a weakness in his disposition that incapacitates him from carrying his nobler purposes into effect. He sees that some particular course of action is his duty, and should be his delight; but his inclinations are fickle and base, and do not conform to his better judgment. The whole moral nature of man is tainted with sin, which prevents him from doing the things he knows to be right.

I venture to offer an explanation of this apparent anomaly, which seems perfectly satisfactory from a scientific point of view. It is neither more nor less than that the development of our nature, under Darwin's law of natural selection, has not yet overtaken the development of our religious civilization. Man was barbarous but yesterday, and therefore it is not to be expected that the natural aptitudes of his race should already have become moulded into accordance with his very recent advance. We men of the present centuries are like animals suddenly transplanted among new conditions of climate and of food: our instincts fail us under the altered circumstances.

My theory is confirmed by the fact that the members of old civilizations are far less sensible than those newly converted from barbarism of their nature being inadequate to their moral needs. The conscience of a negro is aghast at his own wild, impulsive nature, and is easily stirred by a preacher, but it is scarcely possible to ruffle the self-complacency of a steady-going Chinaman.

The sense of original sin would show, according to my theory, not that man was fallen from a high estate, but that he was rapidly rising from a low one. It would therefore confirm the conclusion that has been arrived at by every independent line of ethnological research—that our forefathers were utter savages from the beginning; and, that, after myriads of years of barbarism, our race has but very recently grown to be civilized and religious (p. 327).

Galton was so fond of this passage that he reprinted it, *in toto,* in his autobiography, forty years later.[24] His fondness for it is rather illuminating. Like the overly enthusiastic rhetoric that he had used to describe his plan for a perfect society in the first part of "Hereditary Talent and Character," this passage reveals his emotional attachment to the idea of mental heredity. He had adopted the somewhat agnostic, somewhat petulant, somewhat antagonistic religious stance that was so typical of Victorian scientific intellectuals.[25] Galton appears to have been delighted by the fact that the doctrine of mental heredity provided him with a tool with which to undercut the power of various religious orthodoxies. Perhaps he became committed to the idea of mental heredity not only because of the social programs that could be built around it but also because of the religious creeds that it could destroy.

"Hereditary Talent and Character" contained harbingers of every major contribution that Galton was to make to the sciences of biology, psychology, and statistics, and yet, by even the kindest contemporary estimation, it was not a scientific paper. Its internal logic was a shambles; paragraphs tumbled after one another in no apparent order; sweeping generalizations were presented without proofs; proofs when they were presented did not lead to the conclusions that were drawn from them; topics were introduced, discussed, dropped and then reintroduced several pages and several intervening topics later. "Hereditary Talent and Character" seemed, with good reason, to have fallen on deaf ears. The paper was rarely cited by his contemporaries, and in all the extant Galton correspondence there exists only one letter remarking upon it.[26]

When read as a political rather than a scientific tract "Hereditary Talent and Character" makes more sense. The differential skepticism that is manifested in it, the habit of accepting some ideas and rejecting others for no apparently valid reason, was more acceptable in political discourse than in scientific discourse, even in the nineteenth century. *Macmillan's Magazine* was not the sort of publication one would choose if one were hoping to address a scientific audience; it was a magazine of general cultural and political interest, representing a fairly conservative constituency in 1865.[27] When all this is added together—rambling logic, a somewhat peculiar context for the arguments, evident biases, and placement in a nonscientific journal—it seems fair to read the paper not as a scientific treatise but as the result of an argument that Galton may have been having with himself and with the social theorists of his day.

Francis Galton before 1865

The year 1865 represents something of a watershed in Galton's life. Before 1865 he had pursued various scientific subjects but had had little interest in biology; after 1865, and for the rest of his life, he was obsessed with heredity and associated problems. "Hereditary Talent and Character" had enormous significance for him; of all his writings, and they were many, it is the only one from which he quoted extensively in his autobiography. Almost all of his memorable scientific work evolved from concerns that were first expressed in that paper. And yet, as we have seen, the paper was fundamentally a political tract, and it was dominated by an *idée fixe*—the eugenic principle—which was never again to be far from his mind. Much of Galton's subsequent work on heredity was more consciously "scientific,"—the logic was tighter, the mathematics somewhat more sophisticated, the evidential base somewhat broader, and the argument more clearly directed to the scientific community—but the *idée fixe* was still there. He was committed to the eugenic principle, and it dominated the development of his scientific ideas. He was aware of this and he regarded it as entirely proper, because to him the achievement of a eugenic society was a more important goal than the achievement of scientific truth.[28]

The details of Galton's life before 1865 provide important clues to the source of that *idée fixe*. Francis Galton was, in many ways, a typically idiosyncratic Victorian. Born in 1822, the youngest of seven children of Samuel Tertius Galton, a successful Birmingham banker, and Violetta Darwin Galton, one of the many daughters of Erasmus Darwin, he was, both by birth and by inclination, a member of that small circle of eccentric Englishmen, the Victorian intelligentsia. Both his paternal and maternal grandfathers had been founding members of the Birmingham Lunar Society; Galton considered himself an heir to the scientific and intellectual tradition that that society represented. Grandson of a Quaker, son of a member of the Established Church, he was only a nominal churchgoer and was more often inclined to scoff than to pray. Angered by the "condition of England" and enthused about his own proposals for reform, he tended, more often than not, to vote Conservative. Fellow of the Royal Society, member of the Athenaeum, occasionally secretary of the British Association, he belonged to all the right "clubs" and had all the right friends—Sir Richard Burton, Herbert Spencer, the younger Darwins—to qualify as a member of the intellectual establishment.[29]

As a child Galton was regarded as something of a prodigy; he learned the alphabet at eighteen months, read at two and one-half years, signed his name at three, memorized poetry at five, and discussed the *Iliad* at six. Despite this auspicious beginning his school record was relatively undistinguished. At King Edward's School in Birmingham (The Birmingham Free School) he showed little aptitude for classical studies and chafed at the limitations that were placed upon him, occasionally becoming something of a disciplinary problem. At the age of sixteen, he was removed from school, much to his joy. His parents decided that he should enter the medical profession and he became a pupil at Birmingham General Hospital; for one year he accompanied surgeons on their rounds, assisted in operations and post-mortems, and attended patients in the accident room. The next year (1839) found him enrolled at King's College Medical School in London. Although Galton seems to have flourished at King's (he won the prize in forensic medicine and was second in physiology) he was not entirely satisfied with a medical education and wished to read mathematics at a university. After much discussion, and over much parental objection, he was allowed to proceed to Cambridge (Trinity College) in 1840.

At Cambridge Galton was an active collegian, but his academic record was, once again, undistinguished. Although his circle of friends included some of the most notable scholars of his day, among them H. S. Maine, Henry Hallam, and Frank Lushington, he was never able to equal their success in examinations and prize competitions. It is interesting to note that in his autobiography he made no mention of his academic pursuits at Cambridge, although he devoted considerable space to his social activities during those three years; reading parties, breakfast parties, drinking parties, hiking parties, and dancing parties abounded, but of books and professors there is very little mention. Galton just managed to escape failing his first set of exams (the "Little Go") and subsequently decided that it would be futile to attempt the second-year scholarship examinations. During his third year, while preparing for the final set of exams (the "Honors" exam) he suffered a nervous breakdown and was forced to leave Cambridge with an ordinary degree (a "Poll").

Apparently for want of something better to do he spent a few more terms studying medicine, first at Cambridge and then at St. George's Hospital in London, but his desultory progress toward a medical career was abruptly ended when, in the autumn of 1844, his father died, leaving an enormous inheritance.

Medical studies were quickly abandoned and within a few months, "being much upset and craving for a healthier life,"[30] he set out on a tour of the Middle East. For the next eight years he wandered, first in the Middle East (1845–46), then through Scotland (1846–50), then, under the aegis of the Royal Geographic Society, through parts of South West Africa. There is some indirect evidence that he suffered a good deal of mental anguish during those years, or, at the very least, that he began to question some of his most basic beliefs. The most telling evidence is the fact that almost all his correspondence of these years was destroyed, although his letters from other years were meticulously preserved by his family. Galton was probably thinking of his own experience when, many years later and in a different context, he wrote: "Men are too apt to accept as axiomatic law, not capable of further explanation whatever they see recurring day after day without fail. . . . Travel in distant countries, by unsettling these quasi-axiomatic ideas, restores to the educated man the freshness of childhood in observing new things and in seeking reasons for all he sees."[31]

After returning from Africa in 1852 Galton began to settle down. Within a year and a half he had married and taken up permanent residence in London. His wife, Louisa Butler, was the daughter of the headmaster of Harrow. Despite an active social life after his marriage Galton found time to write an account of his exploration for the Royal Geographic Society (*Tropical South Africa,* 1853) and soon became active on its council. In 1855, after the first British military disasters in the Crimean War, he decided to offer his services to the government and spent the next year giving courses in campaigning to the troops at Aldershot. *The Art of Travel,* a guide for travelers who must rough-it, was published in the same year. At about this time he began to be a familiar figure in London scientific circles. He was elected to the Royal Society in 1856, to the managing board of the Kew Observatory in 1858, to the Royal Statistical Society in 1860, and to the Ethnological Society at about the same time. He published a variety of papers during these years, dealing with such subjects as map making, geographic measurement, geographic instruments, weather prediciton, weather mapping, and cyclonic behavior (having become interested in meteorology as a result of his work at Kew).

After 1860 Galton's scientific interests began to change, but the style of life that he had established for himself during the 1850s remained farily stable. A good part of each year, usually the late spring and summer, was spent traveling, either on the continent or visiting the various branches of the Galton and Butler families in England. Usually these summer excursions were capped by attendance at the British Association meetings early in September. During the winter months his time was divided between his own scientific pursuits and a variety of administrative responsibilities. In 1868 he became one of the initial members of the Meteorological Council, which supervised the activities of the Meteorological Office of the Board of Trade, and remained a member until 1901. Similarly, he remained a member of the Kew Committee (responsible for the administration of Kew Observatory) for forty-three years, serving as chairman for twelve of those years, 1889–1901. Both councils took up a great deal of his time, as did similar duties for the Royal Society (on the council of the Royal Society intermittently between 1865 and 1884) the British Association (sectional chairman three times, and general secretary, 1863–67) and the Anthropological Institute (president, 1885–89).

It is difficult to determine precisely why Galton's scientific interests shifted from the physical to the biological sciences after 1860, but it is perfectly clear that almost all the active research that engaged him during the remainder of his life focused on heredity and attendant problems. The latter part of his career can be divided conveniently into five distinct periods. The first, between 1860 and 1869, was the exploratory stage; during this time he first became aware of what he termed "the heredity doctrine" and its possible use in the reformation of society. *Hereditary Genius* (1869) summarized Galton's researches of this period: his first attempts to prove the predominance of heredity over environment by statistical means, and his various rummagings in the literature of heredity, primarily in Darwin's *Variations of Animals and Plants under Domestication*. During the second period, from 1869 to 1876, he devoted much of his thought to physiological theories of heredity, attempting to establish an experimental proof for pangenesis, and then when this failed, attempting to construct an alternative theory that would fit the experimental evidence. During this period he published *English Men of Science: Their Nature and Nurture* (1874), which, as its title suggests, was another attempt to prove the predominance of heredity over environment, this time specifically in the production of scientific ability.

After 1876 Galton realized that physiological theorizing was probably not his bent and he turned his attention to the development of statistical and anthropometric techniques that might assist his cause. His researches during this period, from 1876 to 1889, were many and varied, ranging from the construction of machines that would test human abilities, to studies of composite portraiture, and to extremely sophisticated statistical analyses of data acquired at the various anthropometric laboratories that he had established during this time. Two books, *Inquiries into Human Faculty* (1883) and *Natural Inheritance* (1889) summarized his work during this period, perhaps the most productive of his career.

After the publication of *Natural Inheritance* Galton discovered that the academic world had become interested in his work. Partially through his own initiative and partially because of the enthusiasm of Karl Pearson and W. F. R. Weldon, a biometric laboratory was founded at University College, London, and Galton gave his first set of academic lectures on variation and correlation. The period between 1889 and 1901 was what one might call a period of consolidation; Galton did not begin any new researches but he, Pearson, Weldon, and others followed up the implications of the work that he had done earlier.

After 1901 the eugenics movement began in earnest. By this time Galton was almost eighty years old and in failing health, but whatever limited energies he still had at his command he devoted to the propagation of the eugenic gospel. He had enunciated his plans for the reformation of society by controlled breeding many years earlier, but in 1901, for the first time, his proposals struck a responsive political chord in the English intelligentsia. The Eugenics Education Society was founded, research fellowships in eugenics were established at University College, London, and, finally, in 1907, a eugenics laboratory was endowed at the same institution. Galton gave public lectures, wrote endless numbers of popular articles, and attended endless numbers of public meetings—all in the hope of furthering the eugenic cause.

By the time of his death in 1911 Galton had been awarded almost every major honor that could be bestowed upon on English man of science: the Darwin-Wallace Medal of the Linnaean Society; honorary degrees at Cambridge and Oxford; the Gold Medal, Darwin Medal, and Copley Medal of the Royal Society; the Huxley Medal of the Anthropological Institute—and finally, a knighthood. He died knowing that he had been the founder of a flourishing political movement as well as the founder of a flourishing tradition of scientific research—biometry. The only disappointment that may have marred his later years was the realization that although he had created eugenics he had not fulfilled his eugenic obligation; scion of two prominent English families, married to the daughter of a third, Galton had had no children.

"Hereditary Talent and Character" is thus a reflection of the idiosyncrasies of its author. The contents of the article probably did not surprise any of his friends at the time, despite the fact that none of his previous work had focused on the problems of human heredity and ethnology. "Hereditary Talent and Character," was, in many ways, a natural extension of Galton's personality and a natural consequence of certain problems that were troubling him at the time the paper was written.

The mathematical format of the first half of the paper is very characteristic of Galton; he was compulsively interested in measuring and counting.[32] Wherever he went and whatever he did, he usually found something to count along the way and he often carried his compulsion to marvelous extremes. While traveling in South Africa, for example, he was overcome by a desire to discover the precise measurements of some hefty Hottentot ladies. "I have dexterously even without the knowledge of the parties concerned, resorted to actual measurement. . . . I sat at a distance with my sextant, and as the ladies turned themselves about, as women always do, to be admired, I surveyed them in every way and subsequently measured the distance of the spot where they stood—worked out and tabulated the results at my leisure."[33] Finding himself bored at a meeting of the Royal Society Galton constructed a small pocket "ticker" and measured the frequency with which various members of the Society were fidgeting in their seats.[34] Finding himself ill and confined at home he decided to determine the precise combination of variables that would produce a perfect cup of tea.

> Feb 15 Tuesday morning. [pot] heated
> to $\frac{178°}{169°}$ [in] four minutes. + $\frac{194°}{186°}$ in seven
> minutes hot and decocted. 2nd cup $\frac{194°}{174°}$
> [in] 11 minutes hot and weak.
> Feb. 16. Evening. $\frac{40m}{48m}$ $\frac{191°}{178°}$ Decoct.
> slightly. Louisa says fresh and little
> body (I have a cold.)[35]

Almost every scientific paper that he had published prior to 1865 was concerned, in some manner, with counting and measurement, whether it be methods of keeping accurate records of weather conditions or methods for determing the accuracy of geographic instruments.

Thus, the fact that Galton used statistical techniques in "Hereditary Talent and Character," and in almost all his subsequent work on heredity, does not necessarily indicate that he had any special perspicacity or genius. While it may be true that in 1865 the sciences of biology and psychology were ripe for quantification, and while it also may be true that Galton's statistical methodology proved fruitful in both sciences, it does not necessarily follow that he realized the power or the relevance of the method that he was adopting. He may well have understood this later on, when he became more fully acquainted with the literature of biology and psychology, but when he first undertook statistical analyses of biographical dictionaries he was simply doing what came naturally to him—measuring and counting. This, then, is the sense in which "Hereditary Talent and Character" represents a natural extension of his personality.

"Hereditary Talent and Character" is also a natural consequence of certain problems that were disturbing Galton in 1864, problems of a political and theological nature. During the thirteen years that separated his return from South West Africa (1852) and the publication of "Hereditary Talent and Character" (1865) Galton was intellectually restless; as he put it, "I was rather unsettled during a few years."[36] A wide variety of subjects piqued his interest momentarily. In the mid-1850s it was geography and campaigning. Later in the 1850s it was instrument-making and testing. In the early 1860s it was meteorology and then ethnology. Intermittently throughout these years he laid plans for new geographical explorations, but his plans were invariably foiled by his own wavering health.[37]

Galton was an accident waiting to happen; a rich and talented man waiting to find some cause (hopefully a scientific one) to which he could commit his overabundant money and energy; a man not simply searching for something interesting to do but for something that would be socially useful. Like so many other wealthy Victorians, especially those who families had been or were dissenters, Galton was not simply content to sit back and enjoy the fruits of his wealth; he felt it was his duty in some way to benefit society. We find indications of this sentiment in a letter, written to him in 1855 by C. J. Anderssen, who had accompanied him on his African expedition and who was, at least for a time, a close friend. Galton had just asked if Anderssen would be interested in joining him at Aldershot, and Anderssen replied: "It was with very great gratification that I learned that you at last had arrived at the goal of your sanguinary wishes. I am sure that your talents and good motives are a sufficient guarantee for the success of the arduous but immensely useful work you are about to embark on.... *By the same wish as yourself to be 'of use in the world'* ... I would gladly try my hand at assisting you to the best of my ability [italics added]."[38] Later, speaking of his disappointment at not being able to undertake additional exploration, Galton reconciled himself to his confinement in England with the thought that "there was an abundance of useful work at home."[39]

In 1865 his search was ended; the utopian scheme that he outlined in "Hereditary Talent and Character"—the scheme that was later called "eugenics"—provided him with a philanthropic cause that could engage all his altruistic and scientific impulses. Conveniently, it also provided a solution to a political problem that had troubled him for many years: by what means, short of revolution, might society be totally reformed? As far back as his student years Galton had been distressed by the "condition of England" (about which almost everyone was distressed in the 1840s) and by the general state of the world. He was not nearly as impressed as some of his Victorian contemporaries were with the achievements of "Progress." Witness this selection from a poem that he wrote at Cambridge in 1843:

> How foolish and how wicked seems the world,
> With all its energies bent to amass
> Wealth, fame or knowledge; scarce a thought
> Of those great voids which this life bridges o'er
> The future and the past eternity,
> Or of that Mighty One who dwelleth here.
> Well may we loathe this world of sin, and strain,
> As an imprisoned dove to flee away;
> Well may we burn to be as citizens
> Of some state, modelled after Plato's scheme.[40]

As another example, here is one of the few extant remnants of his *wanderjahre* correspondence, his own rendition of a passage from Chaucer:

> Fly from the press and dwell with truth
> Suffice unto (be satisfied with) thy good though it be small
> For hoard (hoarding) hath hate and climbing danger

Price (wealth) hath envy and weal is (blinded) deceived by all...
That (which is sent thee) thee is sent receive in buxomness
The wrestling of this world asketh a fall:
Here is no home, here is but wilderness.[41]

During the decade of the 1840s Galton despaired of the condition of the world; during the decade of the 1850s he tried, unsuccessfully, to find a useful role within it. Perhaps, in light of this, we can understand why, during the decade of the 1860s, he fastened with such eagerness upon the idea of human improvement through controlled breeding. The theory of mental heredity provided him with everything that he had been searching for: it was a scientific theory and would require from its proponent further investigations of a scientific character. It was useful, that is to say, though it was a scientific theory it also could be transformed into a practical political program. Above all it was ameliorative; controlled human breeding made possible by the fact of mental heredity was a program that spoke directly to the problem that most concerned Galton—the improvement of the human race.

But why eugenics? Why, of all the possible political programs to which Galton might have been attracted, did he choose this one? Why was he not satisified with the reform movements that were popular in his day, those of the Benthamites or Owenites, for example? Why did he feel it necessary to construct a reform proposal of his own? It is unlikely that we will ever have complete answers to those questions—but incomplete ones may be possible.

From his youth until his old age Galton seems to have favored the Conservative party. At Cambridge he often took the Conservative side in Union debates, and on one occasion, when he chanced to be in the same carriage with a member of the Reform Club, he tried to avoid creating a dispute with the man, but eventually succumbed: "We had a red hot argument... Bessy will, I hope, excuse my not assenting to a radical's ideas."[42] His nephew, Frank Butler, remembers that after 1900 Galton always voted Conservative and was much impressed by Salisbury's prime ministership.[43]

The decade of the 1860s was a time of political and intellectual turmoil in England. The preceding decade had been relatively quiescent—R. K. Webb refers to the 1850s as a period of "consolidation"—but in 1859 signs of turmoil were on the horizon.[44] The international scene was disrupted by a series of disputes—the Italian wars, the American Civil War, the wars between Germany and Denmark, then Germany and Austria—which the English, somewhat to their horror and much to their dismay, could not understand at all. Domestic politics were polarized, occasionally to the point of riot, by the festering sore of franchise reform.

During the 1860s it became fashionable for somewhat conservative intellectuals to express their dissatisfaction with what had been considered the sacred Victorian trinity of ideas: technological progress, political reform, and the superiority of the middle class.[45] John Ruskin, whose *Unto This Last* was published in 1862, and Matthew Arnold, whose *Culture and Anarchy* appeared in 1869, are just two examples of this trend. Although these conservative intellectuals often differed with one another there was one issue on which they commonly agreed; they were adamantly opposed to the principles of political economy.

"Among the delusions which at different periods have possessed themselves of the minds of large masses of the human race, perhaps the most curious—certainly the least creditable—is the modern *soi-disant* science of political economy."[46] According to Arnold, thirty years of Benthamite, Owenite, Cobdenite reform had done nothing more than lower the cultural level of the English people.[47] What good had come of the ethic of progress, conservatives asked. What good had come of the doctrine that all men are created equal at birth and thence made different by environment and education? Political turbulence was as prevalent as it had ever been (witness the events preceding and following the Reform Bill of 1867), the country seemed perpetually on the brink of revolution, poverty had not been abolished and cultural poverty had noticeably increased. True reform would only come about, they maintained, when the basic character of man had changed; legislation had clearly failed to do the job.

Francis Galton shared the convictions of men such as Arnold and Ruskin. He had no fondness for egalitarian ideas and did not hesitate to say so explicitly: "I have no patience with the hypothesis occasionally expressed, and often implied, especially in tales written to teach children to be good— that babies are born pretty much alike and that the sole agencies in creating differences between boy and boy, and man and man are steady application and moral effort. It is in the most unqualified manner that I object to pretensions of natural equality."[48] And certainly, as "Hereditary Talent and Character" demonstrates, he did not believe that past attempts at reform had produced the least improvement in the human race. In fact, and in sympathy with other Victorian conservatives, Galton was convinced that over the years the race had been declining under the influence of improper forms of charity and inheritance; inheritance because it brings great wealth to unfit individuals, and charity because it permits unfit individuals to live, breed, and continue their kind.

Eugenics provided Galton with a safe course between the horns of a dilemma: how to insure that human progress continues (because the ongoing evolution of society requires that man continue to improve), while at the same time not subscribing to naïve egalitarianism, the equality of interests proposed by Bentham and Mill. It is no wonder that Francis Galton, a man who was searching for radical solutions to the social problems of his day but who possessed, nonetheless, very conservative instincts, should have conceived a scheme that vitiated the reformist—egalitarian spirit. Considering the year in which he was writing, 1865—the year in which political pressure for egalitarian franchise reform was coming to a head—and considering the personality of the writer, it is no wonder at all.

Several of Galton's contemporaries understood that his eugenic schemes contradicted the ideas of the political economists; depending upon their own political position they either reproached or applauded him for it. "The Doctrine of Heredity throws a needful light upon the question of national education," said one reviewer. "The delusion, which first appears in Helvetius, that proper education can create genius from any child, is still with us," but he hoped that Galton's work would help to dispel the delusion.[49] According to another reviewer, in Galton's work, "the primitive passions for kindred and race are exalted again to their highest dignity; and thus we call to our aid two powerful emotions *which the last century frowned upon,* but which are yet among the most potent that sway mankind—family pride and patriotism."[50]

No other reviewer described the difference between Galton's views and those of older philosophers better than Frances Power Cobbe:

We used first to think . . . that each of us, so far as our mental and moral parts were concerned, were wholly fresh, isolated specimens of creative Power, "trailing clouds of glory," straight out of heaven. Then came the generation which believed in the omnipotence of education. Its creed was, that you had only to "catch your hare" or your child, and were he or she born bright or dull-witted, the offspring of two drunken tramps, or of a philosopher married to a poetess, it was all the same. It depended only on the care with which you trained it and crammed it with "useful knowledge" to make it a Cato and a Plato rolled into one. . . .

Now it seems we are trotting up to another fence, *videlict,* the doctrine that *all* man's faculties and qualities, physical, mental, moral and religious, have a certain given relation to the conditions of his birth. . . . Our whole theory of the meaning and scope of Education must rise from . . . crude delusions.[51]

And no other commentator summarized the disparity between political economy and the new eugenic creed better than John Stuart Mill: "Of all the vulgar modes of escaping from the consideration of the social and moral influences on the human mind, the most vulgar is that of attributing the diversities of conduct and character to inherent original natural difference."[52] That vulgar idea was, of course, precisely the one that Galton espoused.

Thus Galton was a closer intellectual ally of Ruskin and Arnold than he was of Darwin and Huxley. This fact helps us to understand why he opposed the inheritance of acquired characteristics at a time when almost all reputable biologists, Darwin included, were prone to accept it. He was not a naturalist; on most biological issues he was willing, if not eager, to accept the opinion of more eminent biologists—and there was no opinion that he esteemed more than that of Charles Darwin. Yet on the issue of the inheritance of acquired characteristics Galton stood firmly opposed to Darwin, despite Darwin's repeated efforts to convince him otherwise. Wherever Darwin discussed instances of the inheritance of acquired traits in *The Variation of Plants and Animals under Domestication* Galton placed a skeptical comment or a question-mark in the margin.[53] Galton's "stirp" theory was almost identical to Darwin's pangenesis theory except on one point: in Galton's scheme the inheritance of acquired characters was impossible.[54] When Darwin objected to this and recommended that Galton read Brown-Sequard's articles about the inheritance of acquired epilepsy in guinea pigs, Galton responded by trying to find fallacies in Brown-Sequard's argument.[55] Other biologists were willing to make allowances for Brown-Sequard, but Galton refused.

From a political point of view he had good reasons for doing so; the hypothesis of the inheritance of acquired characters leads to a political stance that Galton found inimical—political economy. Chronologically, his interest in politics predated his interest in biology, and it seems likely that he initially rejected Lamarckian ideas on political grounds alone. It is not surprising, in light of this, that he failed to discuss the biological implications of the continuity of germ plasm in "Hereditary Talent and Character." Not being a naturalist and not fully comprehending the Darwinian theory, he did not realize that the inheritance of acquired characters was an essential part of the theory of evolution by natural selection as first formulated by Darwin in 1859. Galton was willing to accept Darwin's authority on matters biological but not on matters philosophical, and the inheritance of acquired characters was, to Galton, primarily an issue in political philosophy. In this connection it is significant to note that Galton did not suggest that it might be profitable to perform biological experiments on the inheritance of acquired characters until 1889—long after he had convinced himself, on other grounds, that the phenomenon simply did not exist.[56]

The proposals for social reform that Galton first enunciated in "Hereditary Talent and Character" fulfilled his need to play the role of a social philanthropist. The strength of his commitment to the eugenic principle is demonstrated by the tenacity with which he clung to that idea, despite repeated discouragement over the years. Criticism reached him from almost every side. Charles Darwin was less than enthusiastic: "Very many thanks for Fraser: [Galton's article, "Hereditary Improvement,"] greatly interested by your article. The idea . . . is quite new to me, and I should suppose to others. I am not, however, so hopeful as you."[57] Reviewers had a tendency either to ignore the idea or to pass it off as inconsequential: "Though this [the improvement of the human race] is the author's general aim, his book is more interesting in curious detail than valuable for any advice as to the conscious modification of the human race."[58] But Galton persisted. Even after it had become clear that the public was not ready to accept his views about the necessity of planned breeding, he continued privately to dream of a eugenic Utopia—the new social order that would conform to principles of human heredity and would adopt race betterment as an ethical creed.[59] He did not formally reintroduce his eugenic ideas until 1901.[60] At that time he recieved considerable public acclaim and for the remainder of his life was involved in a feverish attempt to establish eugenics as a viable social program. *Biometrika* was founded, the Eugenic Laboratory at University College, London, was financed, fellowships were endowed, pamphlets published, and the Eugenics Education Society established. As early as 1884 G. J. Romanes, a personal friend, had rightly observed that "Mr. Galton is indefatigable in his zeal to promote the cause of eugenics."[61]

The strength of Galton's committment to the eugenic principle was also a function of the theological void that it filled for him. Before 1865 he often questioned the truth of the religious doctrines that he had been taught as a child; these doubts may have been responsible for the nervous breakdown that he suffered in 1842. During the 1840s many young members of the English intelligentsia began to question the faith in which they had been raised. "All around us the intellectual lightships had broken from their moorings and it was then a new and trying experience . . . the lights [were] all drifting, the compasses all awry, and nothing [was] left to steer by but the stars."[62] There is some evidence to indicate that Galton was no exception. In 1843 he was less than enthusiastic about the state of religion:

> The heart of man is intellectualized,
> and the high souls of other days are gone;
> Men in whose noble gait and manly eye
> Was written hardihood to dare the last
> Their life, their wealth, their all, at duty's hest
> Feeling in truth that they but creatures were,
> While their Creator was omnipotent,
> Yet sanctified as temples for his use,
> Wherefore they deeply did respect themselves.
> But these are times of flippant vanity,
> Of self sufficiency, not self-respect,
> Of vain philosophy and arrogance,
> As though the supercilious reasoner
> Were fit material for a christian.
> Oh! would I had the simple earnestness,
> The faith of those unlearned fishermen,
> Who left their nets and followed—all for love.[63]

Not long after writing this poem Galton departed for a tour of the Middle East; his encounters with Mohammedans there may have increased his doubts about

Christianity. He often referred to the purity and righteousness of orthodox Mohammedans; in this respect he thought that they were better men than most Christians. Notice, for example, the rhetorical tone that he used in describing an encounter with an Arabian sheikh:

The Sheikh was sent for, and I shall never forget his entrance. The cabin reeked with the smells of a recent carouse [Galton and his companions had been drinking all night], when the door opened and there stood the tall Sheikh, marked with sand on his forehead that indicated recent prostration in prayer. The pure moonlight flooded the Bacchanalian cabin, and the clear cool desert air poured in. I felt swinish in the presence of his Moslem purity and imposing mien.[64]

Another indication of Galton's religious doubts is the fact that for a span of almost twenty years he was interested in the phenomena of spiritualism. The spiritualism fad, which reappeared sporadically on the English scene during the second half of the nineteenth century, began with the work of an American medium, Daniel Douglas Home.[65] The first report of Home's powers reached England sometime during the early fifties; when he crossed the Atlantic he was entertained by such illustrious Englishmen as Robert Browning, Lord Brougham, Sir David Brewster, and Sir Edward Bulwer Lytton. Many English intellectuals believed that if Home's powers were proven real, the existence of an immortal soul could not be doubted. "The Right Hon. John Bright . . . after expressing the wonder that he felt at Mr. Home's manifestations . . . added cautiously, 'I do not say that this is so, but if it be true, it is the strongest tangible proof we have of immortality'."[66] Many of those who were interested in spiritualism were searching for a religious certainty that they could no longer find in the doctrines of Christiantiy. "We may doubt whether Mr. Bright's share in the earnest conversation has been quite accurately reported; but we may be sure that the words assigned to him might be assigned with perfect truth to a thousand others. . . . Their faith in Moses and the prophets has grown a little doubtful; they are seeking for something nearer and more tangible . . . and they find it in table-turning."[67]

Louisa Galton's diary for the year 1853 contains an addition in her husband's hand that reads, simply, "Spirit-rapping mania."[68] Twenty years later, when Home had again returned to England and spiritualism was once again a fad, Galton began attending seances; his reaction to the mediums was far from skeptical. "I have been twice . . . in a seance with Miss Fox [a disciple of Home's] . . . I can only say, as yet, that I am utterly confounded with the results and I am very disinclined to discredit them."[69] In the 1870s, as in the previous periods of his life, he was much concerned about the question of the existence of a God-given soul, a question to which the phenomena of spiritualism appeared relevant. After attending seances for almost two years, and after Huxley and Darwin had both expressed their disapproval, Galton finally lost faith in the reliability of the mediums.[70] His tenacity on the matter of spiritualism was not unlike his tenacity on the matter of eugenics; both of them spoke to some emotional need deep within.

Galton seems to have adhered to the doctrines of Christianity—although perhaps not entirely enthusiastically—until sometime between 1860 and 1864, when his enthusiasm disappeared and he became, to all intents and purposes, an agnostic. In a letter written to Darwin in 1869 Galton gave *The Origin of Species* a good deal of the credit for his intellectual transformation:

I always think of you in the same way as converts from barbarism think of the teacher who first relieved them from the intolerable burden of their superstition. I used to be wretched under the weight of the old fashioned ''arguments from design'' of which I felt, though I was unable to prove to myself, the worthlessness. Consequently the appearance of your ''Origin of Species'' formed a real crisis in my life; your book drove away the constraint of my old superstition as if it had been a nightmare and was the first to give me freedom of thought.[71]

The most conclusive evidence of Galton's fall from faith is contained in the pages of ''Hereditary Talent and Character.'' He adopted at least three heterodox positions in that paper: he asserted that man's rational faculties were not a gift from God, that mankind had not been cursed with sinfulness since Adam and Eve, and that religious sentiments were nothing more than evolutionary devices to insure the survival of the human species.

Thus, by 1864 Galton had assumed the classic religious stance of a Victorian–Darwinian scientific intellectual. He regarded most traditional religious observance as absurd and would only agree to participate if urged by another member of his family.[72] He maintained that faith in God was an emotional crutch that he was not so weak as to need; speaking of a relative who had just joined the Catholic Church, he remarked, ''It may be a stable guide for emotional natures, but it would be of no service to . . . me.''[73] In a paper written in 1872 he tried to prove that prayer is useless: he demonstrated that persons who are prayed for most frequently—kings, queens, clergymen, etc.—do not thereby lead longer, healthier, or happier lives.[74] Many members of his family were distressed by the paper, but Galton insisted on republishing it in *Inquiries Into Human Faculty* in 1883.[75]

Galton did not think it much mattered which religion an individual adhered to: ''Men lead happy, useful and honest lives under so many forms of belief that I cannot suppose the precise form of belief to be of much importance.''[76] Most religious leaders seemed to him to be hypocritical, narrow-minded, and excessively dogmatic. ''The religious instructor in every creed is one who makes it his profession to saturate his pupils with prejudice.''[77] The chapter entitled, ''Divines'' in *Hereditary Genius* is a case in point; Galton sought to prove that the constitutions of clergymen were generally weaker than those of other men and that as a group they had not contributed greatly to the history of the country.

Like many agnostics of his day, Galton took particular joy in offending the sensibilities of the religious establishment. Writing to Francis Darwin after having read the manuscript version of Charles Darwin's autobiography, Galton commented:

I cannot express how deeply I have been interested by your father's autobiography. . . . As regards the religious part I really see not the slightest reason for misgiving as to its reception by the outside public. Of course it is one blow the more to self-sufficient dogmatism, in showing that a foremost man does not accept it, but so many blows of this sort have been given to it lately, that this can hardly be taken as a serious and new assault. . . . Have you happened to see Herbert Spencer's just published book on Ecclesiastical Institutions!!! If there still exists a service of bell, book and candle, I can fancy all the Bishops in procession performing it over the book and burning it and its author together amidst hordes of anathemas.[78]

Also not unlike many of his contemporaries Galton delighted in poking fun at what he regarded as some of the more ludicrous aspects of revealed truth. "Tyndall's lecture about bacteria was a great success. . . . I conclude from the theory that the physiological reason of immortality in the next life is that there are no Bacteria in the pure air of heaven!—Nothing to cause corruption."[79]

On the whole, he regarded Christianity as an evolutionary phenomenon that had been suited to the condition of society in an earlier day but which should (and would) soon be replaced by a more progressive system (hopefully, eugenics). The last point is especially significant. Galton repeatedly, insistently, and explicitly stated that upon the demise of Christianity the best alternative ethical code would be eugenics. "I take Eugenics very seriously, feeling that its principles ought to become one of the dominant motives in a civilized nation, much as if they were one of its religious tenets."[80] Under such an ethical code false forms of philanthropy, such as charitable aid to the indigent and the disabled, would cease, to be replaced by a philanthropy which is concerned more for the future of the race than for its present condition. Indeed, all behavior in the present would be judged in terms of its effect upon future generations; for this reason, according to Galton, eugenics should be considered the most properly religious of all forms of philanthropic behavior—it cares more for the future of many individuals than it does for the selfish present of just a few.[81]

When speaking of eugenics, Galton very often used phrases that were exactly the opposite of those that he used when speaking of Christianity. Eugenics, he believed, was a "virile creed," Christianity, on the other hand, was preached by those with "poor constitutions." The doctrine of design was "an intolerable burden" and "a superstition," while the doctrine of control-

led human breeding was "hopeful," "full of promise for mankind," and
—above all—"founded on scientific principles."

Galton's dissent from orthodox Christianity was colored by resentment—
resentment that was only barely concealed. Whenever he wrote about religious sentiments or religious persons there was a tone of bitterness, of disappointment, and disillusion in his words. He never spoke of orthodox men as
admirable men. According to Galton, the religious establishment was, of all
social institutions, the one least likely to produce improvement in the human
race.

Eugenics, the doctrine of mental heredity, the notion of continuity of germ
plasm—for Galton these were all darts that could be thrown in the back of the
religious establishment, whips with which to flail dead or dying religious
beliefs. Eugenics would produce a new, non-Christian moral code. Mental
heredity would make the existence of a God-given soul inconceivable. The
continuity of germ plasm would render nonsensical the notion that some
divine element was introduced into the body of man at birth.

Of all the Christian doctrines that disturbed and distressed the rebellious
Darwinian generation, the doctrine of original sin was the single most ma-
ligned.[82]

What is the secret of the profound interest which Darwinism has excited in the minds
and hearts of more persons than dare to confess their doubts and hopes? . . . It removes
the traditional curse from that helpless infant lying in its mother's arms. . . . It lifts
from the shoulders of man the responsibility for the fact of death. . . . If it is true,
woman can no longer be taunted with having brought down on herself the pangs which
make her sex a martyrdom.[83]

Many of those who felt that Darwinian doctrines had transformed their view
of the world spoke—as had Galton—as if the new ideology had freed them
from the burden of a depressing, inhibited, inhumane approach to life. They
spoke and wrote as if Darwin had lifted them from emotional darkness into
light.

A few years ago when . . . I was invited to Down, and when I was walking with him
[Darwin] in his garden, I felt as if I would fain clasp his feet and try to tell him what he
had been to me. At night I well remember lying sleepless for some hours tracking the
steps of my pilgrimage which had begun in an Egypt of Darkness and been able to clear
Wildernesses by his aid. This spiritual effect of a pure scientific generalisation, as I
have known it in myself and in many other minds, is the most significant phenomenon
of this age.[84]

In view of this, it is small wonder that Francis Galton ended "Hereditary
Talent and Character" by proving that the sense of original sin was nothing
more than an evolutionary phenomenon, produced by the disparity between
the progress of civilization and the slower evolution of man. Darwinism had

released Galton from bondage to the doctrine of original sin; that doctrine may have been the source of the "intolerable religious burden" that Galton spoke of when writing to Darwin in 1869. Once he realized that original sin could be explained on evolutionary grounds Galton was "relieved," a weight was taken from his back. Darwinism had put him on the road to emotional release; eugenics assured that he would never have any need to retreat.

Despite their power, the doctrines of eugenics were not complete and sufficient substitutes for Christianity in Galton's mind. They could replace the ethical code that had sprung from religion, but they could not replace the cosmology that Christianity had proferred. The doctrines of eugenics did not speak to such important problems as the nature of the world and of life on earth. Galton found the answers to these questions in a pantheistic doctrine that he adopted sometime between 1860 and 1864. It was expressed in "Hereditary Talent and Character" in one sentence: "We should . . . look on the nature of mankind, and perhaps on that of the whole animated creation, as one continuous system, ever pushing out new branches in all directions, that variously interlace, and that bud into separate lives at every point of interlacement."[85] What began as a single sentence in 1865 later became the foundation of Galton's entire philosophy. He was wont to speak of it in some crucial place in each of his books and articles; it appeared, for example, in the last paragraph of *Hereditary Genius,* in the last paragraph of his autobiography, and in the last paragraph of his article on the statistical efficacy of prayer. The wording that he used in 1869 was perhaps the most complete, and gives us perhaps the greatest insight into the extent to which this pantheism influenced his scientific work: "Nature teems with latent life, which man has large powers of evoking under the forms and to the extent which he desires. We must not permit ourselves to consider each human or other personality as something supernaturally added to the stock of nature, but rather as a segregation of what already existed, under a new shape, and as a regular consequence of previous conditions."[86] The continuity of germ plasm was, to Galton, the physiological mechanism that transmitted the vitalism of the universe. All individuals were part of one great stream of life—the stream of germ plasm.

We may look upon each individual as something not wholly detached from its parent source,—as a wave that has been lifted and shaped by normal conditions into an unknown, illimitable ocean. There is a solidarity as well as a separateness in all humans, and probably in all lives whatsoever; and this consideration goes far, I think, to establish an opinion that the constitution of the living Universe is a pure theism, and that its form of activity is what may be called co-operative.[87]

Thus, the stream of germ plasm was the tie that linked individuals and the raison d'être for cooperation between individuals, be they mice or men. Each individual, past or present, was part of every other individual—and was therefore responsible to him. Eugenics was the most philanthropic guide to society, because it fully expressed the tie between present and future generations.

It points to the conclusion that all life is single in its essence, but various, ever varying, and inter-active in its manifestations, and that men and all other living animals are active workers and sharers in a vastly more extended system of cosmic action than any of ourselves, much less of them, can possibly comprehend. It also suggests that they may contribute, more or less unconsciously, to the manifestation of a far higher life than our own, somewhat as—I do not propose to push the metaphor too far—the individual cells of one of the more complex animals contribute to the manifestation of its higher order of personality.[88]

These cosmological convictions were the source of Galton's unique approach to biological problems. The Greeks had sought the source of "vital power" in the fluids of the body. In more modern times Haller and Bichat had turned to the study of the tissues of the body in an effort to define the nature of life. Virchow believed that the building-block of life was the cell. Claude Bernard believed that the secret of life lay in the adaptive responses of the organism. Galton was one of the first to believe that the crucial material for the study of life was the material that passed from parent to child in the process of generation, the germ plasm.

Galton and Darwin

Francis Galton was Charles Darwin's first cousin. This fact was undoubtedly significant to Galton during his lifetime and it remains significant to historians today. That the author of *Hereditary Genius* was related to one of the greatest geniuses of his day was not a coincidence. Interpreting the development of Galton's eugenic ideas in terms of his own familial heritage is a temptation that is hard to resist. Similarly, it is tempting to interpret the development of his biological ideas—about particulate or nonparticulate inheritance, about continuous or discontinuous variation, about the role of heredity in evolution by natural selection—as if they derived from Darwin's ideas on the same subjects.

Both these temptations are worth resisting. Galton's genealogy could not have been far from his mind as he worked out his eugenic ideas, but the origins of eugenics were, as we have seen, much more complex than that. By the same token his biological ideas were not simply derived from Darwin's. Galton was influenced by Darwin, but his biological ideas developed in response to imperatives that were uniquely his own and that were, in at least one important instance, totally at variance with Darwin's.

Galton and Darwin were first cousins who were almost a generation apart in age; Darwin was born in 1809 and Galton in 1822. Before 1869 they seem to have had little contact. There are only five extant letters between Galton and Darwin that predate the year 1869.[89] Galton's engagement diaries do not contain a single reference to trips to Down or visits from the Down family; neither do Louisa Galton's annual accounts of the years 1853–65.[90] In July 1853 Darwin wrote to Galton to congratulate him on the publication of *Tropical South Africa* and to suggest that they might try renewing their acquaintance, but the suggestion seems never to have been taken up.[91] Galton sent copies of his earliest books to Darwin (*Tropical South Africa* and *The Art of Travel*), but neither book appears to have been read carefully. *Tropical South Africa* has none of Darwin's characteristic marks and notes in it; *The Art of Travel* has only two.[92]

Before 1869 Darwin and Galton had very few interests in common, for Galton was not, by any stretch of the imagination, a naturalist. After reading the *Origin of Species* Galton felt as if he had "been initiated into an entirely new province of knowledge."[93] *Tropical South Africa* did not contain a single comment or observation about indigenous plants, animals, or humans; it was almost solely concerned with geography. *The Art of Travel* was just what its title suggests, a practical guide to roughing-it. In the years preceding the publication of the *Origin* there would have been very little reason for Darwin to have sought the ideas and opinions of his younger cousin. Conversely, Galton probably would not have been very interested in Darwin during those years, as he was kept busy by his work at Kew Observatory, his administrative tasks for the Royal Geographic Society, and his extremely active social life in London and on the continent.

Not being a naturalist Galton was in no position to appreciate the significance of the species problem or to comprehend the powerful fashion in which his cousin attempted to solve it. Although Galton repeatedly stated that the *Origin of Species* had made a great impression on his life, it must have done so only in retrospect, for his initial reaction to the book was pedestrian in the extreme. Galton wrote to Darwin: "I hear you are engaged in a second Edition. There is a trivial error in p. 68 about Rhinocerous, which I thought I might as well point out and have taken advantage of the same opportunity to scrawl down a dozen other notes which may or may not be worthless to you."[94] Galton's made four marginal notes in his copy of the first edition of the *Origin:* three of them were pencil lines demarcating certain passages in the text; the fourth, characteristically enough, was a rough calculation of the rate of population increase from one original pair.[95]

Galton never really understood the argument for evolution by natural selection, nor was he interested in the problem of the creation of new species. In *Hereditary Genius* (1869) he made his first attempt to analyze the Darwinian theory; anyone familiar with Darwin's work will immediately recognize a gross misinterpretation. "It is shown by Mr. Darwin, in his great theory of *The Origin of Species* that all forms of organic life are in some sense convertible into one another, for all have, according to his views, sprung from common ancestry, and therefore A and B having both descended from C, the lines of descent might be remounted from A to C, and redescended from C to B."[96] Darwin had never maintained that the evolutionary process could be reversed, and he had certainly never said that all forms of organic life are interconvertible.

Even after Galton had been involved in heredity studies for almost twenty years he still was unable to come to grips with the doctrine of natural selection. In 1886 he conceived the idea of erecting a monument to Erasmus Darwin in Litchfield Cathedral and proposed that the placque should read:

> In memory of
> Erasmus Darwin, M.D. F.R.S.
> Physician, Philosopher and Poet.
> Earliest propounder of the Theory
> elaborated by his more distinguished grandson
> Charles Darwin
> which ascribes to the operation of animals and plants
> prompted in the first instance by their individual needs
> the secondary and higher function
> of modifying through inheritance
> by various indirect and slow though certain methods
> in increasing adaptation
> to the habits of each other and to their physical surroundings
> and thus of furthering
> the development of organic nature as a whole.

Galton sent this text to a number of persons who might be interested in sponsoring the monument. One copy went to Thomas Huxley. Huxley's reply was quick and to the point: the ideas of Erasmus Darwin and his more distinguished grandson do not resemble each other, he said, and then added a review of the basic principles of Darwinism for Galton's benefit. Galton graciously accepted Huxley's criticism; "I see that the proposed epitaph on Dr. Erasmus Darwin must be wholly abandoned," and in its final version the epitaph was indeed much changed:

> Erasmus Darwin, M.D. F.R.S.
> A skillful observer of Nature
> vivid in imagination, indefatigable in research
> original and far-sighted in his views.
> His speculations were mainly directed to problems

which were afterwards more successfully solved by his Grandson
Charles Darwin
an inheritor of many of his characteristics.[97]

Not being a naturalist, and not being conerned about the species problem, Galton was not a member of that select group whom Darwin had consulted before the publication of the *Origin*. When Darwin wrote to Hooker in March 1860 to present a list of naturalists who had become converts to the doctrine of natural selection, Galton's name was not on the list.[98] Even after the publication of "Hereditary Talent and Character" in 1865, contact between Galton and Darwin did not noticeably increase. No correspondence is extant for those years, despite the fact that Darwin had read, at least cursorily, both of Galton's articles.

This cool relationship between Galton and Darwin began to change after 1869, largely as a result of Galton's reaction to the publication of Darwin's *The Variations of Animals and Plants Under Domestication* (1868). Galton fastened upon this book with remarkable zeal; if his reaction to his cousin's first book had been somewhat pedestrian and casual, his reaction to the second was just the opposite—informed, concerned, and intense. Galton was searching for illumination on the subject of heredity. He made very few marks in the first volume of Darwin's book—which dealt with variation—but Volume II is full of penciled notes. The first three chapters on "Inheritance" and the last two on "Pangenesis" are the most heavily marked of all.[99] These notes indicate that by 1868 Galton had formed very concrete ideas about heredity. He had a distinct point of view and a distinct idea of the additional information that he wanted.

In 1868, as in 1865, Galton was still skeptical of the inheritance of acquired characteristics. For example, where Darwin had written, "In all such cases . . . in which the parent has had an organ injured on one side, and more than one child has been born with the same organ affected on the same side, the chances against mere coincidence are enormous,"[100] Galton underlined the words, "mere coincidence are enormous," and scribbled in the margin, "He might have had an infirm organ to begin with or if not he, his wife, or his wife's family must have." Where Darwin had spoken approvingly of Brown-Sequard's experiments on the inheritance of acquired epilepsy in guinea pigs, Galton wrote, "This is not conclusive."[101]

By 1868 Galton had begun to make a distinction between "inheritance" and "acquired characters," two terms that Darwin often considered under the same head. Galton had a skeptical reaction whenever Darwin wrote of the latter, but he had a favorable reaction whenever Darwin indicated the wide-ranging effects of the former. For example, where Darwin had written, "In some few cases, in which both parents are similarly characterized, inheritance seems to gain so much force by the combined action of the two parents, that it counteracts its own power and a new modification is the result,'' Galton indicated his approval with an exclamation mark in the margin.[102] Contrarily, where Darwin had commented that, ''There is a considerable body of evidence showing that even mutilation, and the effects of accidents, specially or perhaps exclusively when followed by disease are occasionally inherited. There can be no doubt that the evil effects of long continued exposure in the parent to injurious conditions are sometimes transmitted to the offspring.''[103] Galton had appended a mute but significant comment of his own: ''?''. When Darwin used the word ''inheritance'' he intended to denote, among other things, hereditary characters that had been acquired during the life of the parent. Galton apparently objected to this definition; he had decided that acquired characters did not properly belong under that heading. What had begun as a sociological intuition in 1865 had become by 1868 a biological conviction.

Galton's marginal notes in *The Variations* ... also indicate that he had reacted favorably to the theory of pangenesis that was presented in the last chapters of the book. Despite his reservations about the inheritance of acquired characters (which was hypothetically possible under the theory) Galton liked pangenesis because it was potentially mathematisable and because it corresponded to his metaphysical presumptions about the way the universe should be.

While reading the chapters on pangenesis Galton had frequently translated Darwin's prose into mathematics. Where, for example, Darwin had written, ''There is a latent tendency in all pigeons to become blue, and, when a blue pigeon is crossed with one of any other color, the blue tint is generally pre-potent,'' Galton wrote in the margin:

> a is blue and red
> b is blue and black
> the offspring a_2^{+b} is blue
> and ½ red and ½ black in which
> case the blue may well be prepotent.[104]

Galton explored some of the ways in which pangenesis might be mathematised in *Hereditary Genius*. ''The theory of Pangenesis,'' he said, ''brings all the influences that bear on heredity into a form that is appropriate for the grasp of mathematical analysis.''[105] The mathematical analysis that he had in mind was not sophisticated. An individual, he said, would be composed of gemmules of two sorts: the first (Gr—where r was a fraction smaller than one) was derived unchanged from his ancestors, and the second ($G[1-r]$) was modified through individual variation. The contribution of ancestors to the nth degree would be $Gr^{n+1}+G[r^n - r^{n+1}]$. Having derived this expression Galton was not quite sure what might be done with it; there were no real numbers to plug into the formula. Those missing constants, he thought, might someday be supplied, "through averages of facts, like those contained in my tables," by which he meant the statistical analyses of bio-graphical dictionaries that he had presented in earlier chapters of the book.[106] Thus, Galton liked pangenesis because it was quantifiable and because it might make use of the sort of statistics that he loved to pursue.

There was, in addition, something about pangenesis that appealed to Galton's vision of the universe in which all living things are continuous and connected by some material agent. Darwin's gemmules might well be the physical agents of continuity in the great chain of life. "Nature teems with latent life, which man has large powers of evoking under the forms . . . which he desires," Galton wrote, in *Hereditary Genius*. He imagined a great sea of gemmules that would violate time by connecting each generation to the next: "We may look upon each individual as something not wholly detached from its parent source, as a wave that has been lifted and shaped by normal condi-tions in an unknown, illimitable ocean."[107] Galton did not say that pangenesis might be a new type of pantheism, but by juxtaposing his discussion of gemmules with a discussion of "the Universe as a pure theism" he made his implication rather clear.[108]

Thus, the theory of pangenesis appealed to several levels of Galton's in-tellect. He liked it, on the most superficial level, because it explained and recognized the phenomena of heredity. The fact that it had been proposed by his illustrious cousin must have added to its attractiveness. Pangenesis was potentially mathematisable and it corresponded, perhaps almost in a subcon-scious way, to Galton's metaphysical instincts. The only quibble that he might have had with pangenesis was on the issue of the inheritance of acquired characters. In subsequent years when he tried to modify the theory it was just this feature that he sought to expunge.

Hereditary Genius was published in November 1869. At the end of De-cember Darwin sent Galton an enthusiastic congratulatory letter; "I do not think I ever in all my life read anything more interesting and original."[109] Twelve days earlier Galton had written to Darwin to ask advice about begin-ning some experiments that would test pangenesis.[110] With this exchange of letters the cool relationship between Galton and Darwin came to an end.

Charles Darwin was quite attached to the theory of pangenesis, despite the fact that the scientific world had not greeted it with much enthusiasm. Huxley and Hooker, Darwin's closest scientific advisers, had been more than mildly skeptical. Reviewers in the learned journals had been openly and positively critical. Darwin remained convinced that he was right and that subsequent generations would bear out his contention: "Although my hypothesis of pangenesis has been reviled on all sides, yet I must still look at generation under this point of view.''[111] He sincerely believed in pangenesis, and chided Hooker: ''It is a comfort to me to think that you will be surely haunted on your death-bed for not honouring the great god Pan.''[112]

Darwin was defensive about pangenesis and he encouraged anyone who proposed experiments that might vindicate his position. Francis Balfour and George John Romanes both began their scientific careers in this fashion; they pursued experiments on pangenesis, under Darwin's constantly watchful eye, for several years.[113] Francis Galton did the same, and although he was not a young man when he first proposed his pangenesis experiments (in 1869 Galton was forty-seven) Darwin watched over him as if he were a scientific novice.

What Galton proposed to do was simple in theory but difficult in practice. Darwin had hypothesized that the gemmules would circulate freely after being released by their parent cells throughout the body. If this were the case, Galton reasoned, it might be possible to produce mongrels by injecting blood from one strain into the circulatory system of another and permitting the latter to breed. The experimental difficulties were several. First Galton had to find a breed of animals that was relatively stable and that bred with some frequency. He solved this problem with Darwin's assistance, settling upon a breed of rabbits, silver-grays, whose tendenices to mongrelism were very slight. Then Galton had to determine precisely how much blood would have to be transfused in order to alter the gemmule makeup of an individual rabbit. The third difficulty, perhaps the most insurmountable of all, was the fact that after a transfusion operation was performed the rabbits were often too weak to breed successfully.

Darwin eagerly awaited the results of the experiments; for almost a year Galton kept him constantly informed of their progress. On 15 March 1870: ''I grieve to say that my most hopeful doe was confined prematurely by 3 days having made no nest and all we knew of the matter was finding blood about the cage and the *head* of one of the litter.''[114] Two months later, on May 12th: ''Good rabbit news. One of the latest litters has a white forefoot. . . . The mother was injected from a gray and white and the father from a black and white.''[115] (The white foot, it later turned out, is a normal variant in rabbits of solid color.) On June 25th another twist: ''A curious and, it may be, very interesting result delays my transfusion experiments. It is that 2, and I think all 3, of the does that had been coupled with the largely transfused bucks prove *sterile*. Of course the sterility may be due to constitutional shock, or other minor matters, but, it *suggests* the idea that the reproductive elements are in the portion of the blood which I did *not* transfuse—to wit the fibrine.''[116]

In July the Galtons departed for a European tour; as soon as they returned in October the experiments were resumed. By mid-winter 124 offspring in twenty-one litters had been born and not a single mongrel had appeared. At a meeting of the Royal Society, 30 March 1871, Galton reported his experiments and confessed, somewhat to his dismay, that the results had been entirely negative. "The conclusion from this large series of experiments is not to be avoided, that the doctrine of Pangenesis, pure and simple, as I have interpreted it, is incorrect."[117]

Darwin's reaction to Galton's report was uncharacteristic; he behaved badly. Galton was publicly admonished for having unwittingly misinterpreted his cousin's theory. "In my chapter on Pangenesis in my 'Variations of Animals and Plants Under Domestication,'" Darwin wrote in a letter to *Nature,* "I have not said one word about the blood, or about any fluid proper to any circulating system. It is, indeed, obvious that the presence of gemmules in the blood can form no necessary part of my hypothesis; for I refer in illustration of it to the lowest animals, such as the Protozoa which do not possess blood or any vessels."[118]

Darwin was nit-picking; he had never used the word "blood," but he had implied it when he wrote, "The gemmules . . . must be thoroughly diffused; nor does this seem improbable considering their minuteness, and the steady circulation of fluids throughout the body."[119] Is there a fluid other than blood that circulates steadily throughout the body of complex organisms? During the entire year in which Galton had conducted his experiments Darwin had cooperated fully, and had never hinted at the possibility that the experiments might not be conclusive, not, that is, until after the results had been published.

Galton's forbearance in the face of Darwin's betrayal was truly remarkable. His reply to Darwin, printed in *Nature* the following week, was a model of restraint and humility. He apologized for having misunderstood Darwin's phrasing and respectfully suggested that certain sentences should be changed in the second edition of *Variations.* Galton clothed his dismay at Darwin's behavior in allegory:

For my part, I feel as if . . . having heard my trusted leader utter a cry, not particularly well articulated, but to my ears more like that of a hyena than any other animal, and seeing none of my companions stir a step, I had, like a loyal member of the flock, dashed down a path of which I had happily caught sight, into the plain below, followed by the approving nods and kindly grunts of my wise and most-respected chief. And I now feel, after returning from my hard expedition, full of information that the suspected danger was a mistake, for there was no sign of a hyena anywhere in the neighborhood. I am given to understand for the first time that my leader's cry had no reference to a hyena down in the plain, but to a leopard somewhere up in the trees; his throat had been a little out of order—that was all. Well, my labor has not been in vain; it is something to have established the fact that there are no hyenas in the plain, and I think I see my way to a good position for a look out for leopards among the branches of the trees. In the meantime, *Vive Pangenesis.*[120]

"Approving nods and kindly grunts" scarcely conveys the enthusiasm and concern that Darwin had manifested in his correspondence with Galton during the previous year, but Galton chose to leave it at that.

Galton continued the rabbit experiments for another year and a half after this incident, once again under Darwin's supervision. For a few months during the summer of 1872, while Galton and his wife were traveling on the continent, Darwin took charge of the rabbits at his home in Down. All was to no avail; no matter what improvements were made in the technique of transfusion none of the offspring were mongrelized. Much discouraged, Darwin wrote to Galton in November 1872: "Do you want one more generation? If the next one is as true as all the others, it seems to me superfluous to go on trying."[121] Galton agreed, and within one month the experiments were terminated. "The experiments have, I quite agree, been carried on long enough."[122]

With this letter the active period of communication between Galton and Darwin came to a close. During the remaining ten years of Darwin's life (he died in 1882) only a few letters seem to have been exchanged between the two men, and there was, rather often, a gap of a year or more in their correspondence.[123] In 1873 Darwin wrote to Galton to ask a question about statistics— "If I had 50 men of 2 different nations, and for some reason could not measure all, if I picked out the 10 tallest of each nation, would their mean heights probably give an approximate mean between all 50 of each nation?"[124] Two years later Galton wrote to Darwin to ask a favor—"George [Darwin's son] told me that you would very kindly have some sweet-peas planted for me, and save me the produce."[125] Galton sent Darwin reprints of his published articles and Darwin sent Galton copies of his most recent books.

On one occasion this desultory correspondence regained the tempo that it had had during the transfusion experiments—just prior to the publication of Galton's 1875 paper, "A Theory of Heredity."[126] Darwin wrote to Galton to caution him against using some newly published embryological theories, which (Darwin said) Huxley regarded as dubious.[127] Galton answered the following day and attempted to summarize the contents of his paper. Darwin was unable to follow Galton's summary and asked to see a copy of the article; this was duly sent but Darwin found it no easier to understand. In the succeeding correspondence, Galton tried to clarify his position (which differed from Darwin's on the issue of the inheritance of acquired characters) and Darwin tried to indicate both the source of his confusion and the reasons for his disapproval. In the end Galton found no reason to modify his views (or at least if he did modify them he never said so publicly) and Darwin remained unconvinced, though willing to apologize for his overly harsh criticism. "You are a real Christian," he wrote to Galton, "if you do not hate me for ever and ever."[128]

Such was the nature of the intellectual collaboration between Francis Galton and his cousin; they brushed against each other, but neither course was seriously deflected. Galton may have succeeded in convincing Darwin that hereditary influence on mental development was of some importance, but he certainly never swung Darwin over to a belief in complete hereditary determination. Neither was he able to alter Darwin's convictions about the inheritance of acquired characters. Galton provided Darwin with essential scraps of information—about statistical methods, or about the characteristics of twins, about the habits of South African natives, or about the noncirculation of pangenetic gemmules—but he had no ideological effect upon his cousin whatsoever.

Similarly, Darwin provided Galton with a few essential ideas—"ideas for ideas" to use Bateson's apt phrase—but Galton constructed an entirely different edifice with them. From the *Origin of Species* Galton took the idea of struggle for survival, combined it with a set of convictions about hereditary mental ability, and produced a social theory that Darwin could not entirely approve.[129] From *Variations* Galton took the idea that each organic unit (or cell) in the body develops out of a corresponding germ (or gemmule), but he combined this with the noninheritance of acquired characters and produced a theory of heredity that was, as we shall see, inimical to Darwin's. Thus, Darwin was to Galton as a garden supply shop is to a landscape architect: the shop provides a large selection of seeds and seedlings from which a garden can be grown, but the choice of seeds is made totally by the architect, as are all the decisions about arrangements and combinations of plants. The architect's decisions are determined by his own vision of what a particular site requires. So it was with Galton and Darwin; Galton chose seeds of ideas—one might almost say he picked Darwin's brain—but he combined them, nurtured them, and eventually arranged them into a set of theories that were characteristically and uniquely his own.

Pangenesis and Stirp

Galton's heredity theory was inspired by pangenesis, but it was really pangenesis transmuted. Pangenesis was an *ad hoc* hypothesis, created in order to solve certain problems that were inherent in the theory of evolution by natural selection; it conformed to Darwin's vision of the way heredity had to be. Galton's heredity theory—the stirp theory—was also an *an hoc* hypothesis, but it was created to solve problems that were somewhat different from Darwin's.

From Darwin's point of view a theory of heredity had to explain the following phenomena: (1) inheritance, the fact that like tends to reproduce like; (2) individual variation, the fact that offspring never precisely resemble each other or their parents; (3) directed variations, those variations in a species which, according to Darwin, were due to the accumulated effects of slow environmental change; (4) reversion, the fact that a character often skips one or several generations; (5) the orderly and sequential processes of development and growth, what we would call "embryological development"; (6) the fact that many different modes of reproduction exist in the animal and vegetable kingdoms; and (7) the inherited effects of the use and disuse of organs.[130] For Darwin, each phenomenon had a necessary ontological status. If each phenomenon did not exist the mechanism of natural selection would not solve the problem of evolution. Pangenesis provided a reasonable explanation for each of the phenomena, thereby allowing Darwin to assert their reality.

Francis Galton had no need to make such an assertion. The theory of evolution by natural selection was *prima facie* evident to him (had not his illustrious cousin proposed it?) and did not need to be bolstered by physiological hypotheses. What Galton sought was something different: a physiological mechanism for heredity that would insure the inheritance of all physical and mental characteristics, a mechanism that would, in a sense, make heredity omnicompetent. For this reason Galton's heredity theory had to differ from Darwin's in one crucial feature: environmental effects had to be eliminated. If heredity was omnicompetent, then environment could not influence heredity and acquired characters could never be passed from one generation to the next.

By 1872 Galton had worked out a physiological theory that satisfied this condition.[131] In the original pangenesis theory Darwin had suggested that some gemmules might remain latent, skipping a generation or two. Galton extended the idea of latency to include not some, but all of the hereditary determinants. He suggested that there might be two streams of gemmules: one which was expressed in the adult organism and another which would remain latent in the germinal cells. The latent stream would be passed on, undisturbed, to the next generation. The gemmules would segregate twice: once immediately after fertilization, when the embryonic elements (those that will develop into the adult organism) would diverge from the latent elements, and once again, just before reproduction, when the latent elements would divide in two, one part to be passed on to the next generation, one part to die with the individual. The first segregation would be conducted under a principle of "class representation"; one determinant for each unit of the body would be chosen. The second segregation would be "family representation"; determinants representing each familial strain would be selected (see Fig. 1).

Galton was convinced that his theory was better than Darwin's, despite the fact that, for the moment, he could not explain precisely how such complex segregations might occur. Anything that Darwin could explain, Galton could explain better. Reversion was simply the reappearance of previously latent

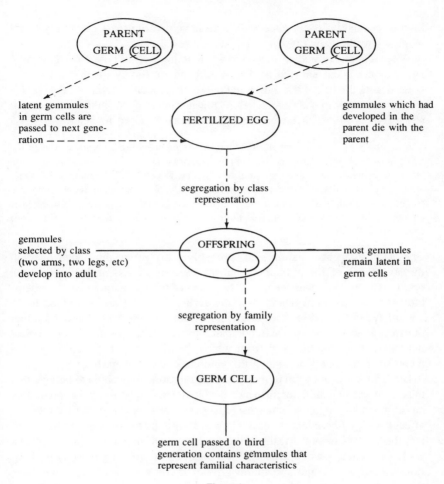

PARENT
GERM CELL

PARENT
GERM CELL

latent gemmules
in germ cells are
passed to next gene-
ration — — — — — — — — →

FERTILIZED EGG

gemmules which had
developed in the
parent die with the
parent

segregation by class
representation

gemmules
selected by class
(two arms, two legs, etc)
develop into adult

OFFSPRING

most gemmules
remain latent in
germ cells

segregation by family
representation

GERM CELL

germ cell passed to third
generation contains gemmules that
represent familial characteristics

Figure 1

gemmules. Individual variation was due to the improbability of two segregations by family representation producing precisely the same set of gemmules.
Development and growth were explained, just as Darwin had explained them,
by the elective affinities of the gemmules one to another. Inheritance was
easier to understand (Galton thought) under his theory than under Darwin's.
The continued appearance of any single character from one generation to the
next was the result of certain statistical probabilities. Given any particular
taxonomic character (the presence of mammary glands, for example) the
chances of its reappearance in each generation would be very high if the
number of determinants for that character in the gemmule pool was also very

high (presumably, every ancestor would have contributed a mammary gland gemmule to the gene pool).

When Galton turned to consider whether his two hypothetical gemmule streams, the latent and the patent, would remain totally distinct from each other during the life of the individual the really crucial difference between his theory and Darwin's appeared. Here the problem of the inheritance (latent stream) of acquired characteristics (patent stream) raised its head.

The two processes are not wholly distinct; on the contrary the embryo, and even the adult in some degree, must receive supplementary contributions derived from . . . the latent elements, because ancestral qualities indicated in early life frequently disappear and yield place to others. *The reverse process is doubtful;* it may exist in the embryonic stage, but it certainly does not exist in a sensible degree in the adult stage, else the later children of a union would resemble their parents more nearly than the earlier ones [italics added].[132]

The latent elements, Galton said, probably reinvigorate the patent ones all during the life of the individual, but the reverse process probably does not occur. His rationale was feeble: "The later children of a union would resemble their parents more nearly than the earlier ones." Had he wanted to he could have destroyed his own argument by simply assuming that the number of patent elements was so small compared to the latent ones that, for statistical purposes, the gemmule pool from which the elder children were born was identical to the one from which the younger children were born.

But Galton did not want to make that assumption. He wanted to believe that the patent stream could not influence the latent stream; he wanted to prove that environmentally induced changes (changes in the patent stream) could not affect heredity (the latent stream). He was struggling to construct a physiological theory that would invalidate the inheritance of acquired characters. His goal, as always, was eugenics: "I am desirous of applying these considerations to the intellectual and moral gifts of the human race. . . . It has been thought by some that the fact of children frequently showing marked individual variation in ability from that of their parents is a proof that intellectual and moral gifts are not strictly transmitted by inheritance. My arguments lead to exactly the opposite result."[133]

Between 1872 and 1875 Galton elaborated upon the points that he had made in "Blood Relationship." "Hereditary Improvement" (January 1873) dealt with social control of breeding and how it could be made palatable.[134] "The History of Twins" (1875) was an attempt to provide statistical evidence for the superiority of nature over nurture.[135] *English Men of Science* (1874) focused on the same theme: Galton circularized the members of the Royal Society and asked them to evaluate the significance of hereditary influences in their lives.[136] Not surprisingly his conclusions about twins and about scientists were markedly alike: "There is no escape from the conclusion that nature prevails enormously over nurture."[137]

In a paper published late in 1875, "A Theory of Heredity," he tried to refine and systematize the views that he had first expressed in 1872.[138] "A Theory of Heredity" differs from "Blood Relationship" only in being less difficult to understand.

The theoretical position stated in both papers was essentially the same, but in the later paper the vocabulary and the point of departure had been somewhat altered. Gone were such awkward expressions as "structureless element" and "familial representation"—replaced by words and phrases that were equally vague, but perhaps more familiar to biological readers: "germ," "gemmule," "struggle for survival," and "organic unit."[139] To simplify matters, Galton invented a word of his own, "stirp"—from the Latin for "root"; stirp denoted the entire pool of germs from which the patent and latent elements arose, the entire pool of germs that was contained in the fertilized egg.

"Blood Relationship" focused on the question, "How are we to understand the relationship that exists between parents, grandparents, great-grandparents and offspring?" "A Theory of Heredity" took a more orthodox tack; its format was very close to the one that Darwin had used in *The Variations. . . .* The main phenomena of heredity were first of all defined, then the main postulates of the "theory of organic units" were outlined, then a new corollary was added—the existence of latent and patent germ streams—and then Galton tried to prove that the stirp theory could provide a better explanation for the phenomena than any theory previously proposed.

"A Theory of Heredity" stimulated a spate of correspondence between Darwin and Galton. Darwin had read an earlier version of the paper and found large parts of it objectionable.[140] In particular, Darwin did not like the passages in which Galton had cast doubt upon the inheritance of acquired characters. In reference to one passage, he wrote, "If this implies that many parts are not modified by use and disuse during the life of the individual, I differ from you, as every year I come to attribute more and more to such agency." Where Galton had said that cases of the inheritance of mutilations were exceedingly rare, Darwin commented, "Such cases can hardly be spoken of as very rare, as you would say if you had received half the number of cases which I have."[141]

The correspondence between Galton and Darwin about "A Theory of Heredity" continued for almost two months. Galton repeatedly tried to explain his position to Darwin and Darwin raised a series of quibbles.[142] During these months Galton revised his paper. He added some paragraphs, but none of them were designed to make his position more palatable to Darwin. In fact his criticism of pangenesis was hardened by the addition of two paragraphs that made his objections to the theory more explicit.[143] None of the offending passages about the inheritance of acquired characters were changed in the least. The section on the meaning and causes of sexuality was even bolder than it had been before.[144]

"A Theory of Heredity" was Galton's last attempt to solve the physiological problem of heredity. After 1875 his thoughts turned from physiology to statistics, from the mechanism to the phenomena of heredity. Perhaps Galton despaired of finding a physiological solution to the problem, or perhaps—and this seems even more likely—he dropped the physiological pursuit of heredity because he was sure he had reached his goal. Galton was not the sort of person to insist, once having found a satisfactory hypothesis, that it had to be tested by experiment; experiment was not his scientific bent. Stirp satisfied him, that was enough; he rarely mentioned it again.

Stirp theory is almost identical to the modern concept of continuity of germ plasm. In 'Blood Relationship" and in "A Theory of Heredity" Galton said, quite explicitly, that once the inheritance of acquired characters was denied the continuity of germ plasm would follow as a logical consequence. "We cannot now fail to be impressed with the fallacy of reckoning inheritance in the usual way, from parents to offspring, using those words in their popular sense of visible personalities. The span of the true hereditary link connects . . . not the parent with the offspring, but the primary elements of the two, such as they existed in the newly impregnated ova, whence they were respectively developed."[145] We have changed some of the words: "latent element" has become "chromosome," "patent element" has become "cytoplasm," "familial and class segregations" have become "mitosis and meiosis," but the substance of the theory remains as Galton left it.

August Weismann, whose name is usually associated with the theory of the continuity of germ plasm, first enunciated his version of the theory on 1883.[146] Galton's theory was virtually identical to Weismann's in most essentials and it was explicated at least a decade earlier. Yet Galton never claimed priority for the discovery, not even after Weismann had, himself, acknowledged Galton's precedence.[147] Galton appears to have forgotten his own work. His autobiography does not mention the papers on stirp and the theory was not mentioned in *Natural Inheritance* either, despite the fact that the book contained a chapter entitled "Processes in Heredity."[148] Either Galton had not fully internalized the scientific ethos that makes priority in discovery a matter of deep concern, or he simply did not regard the stirp theory as terribly important.

The latter seems more likely to be the case. Stirp theory was closely linked to eugenics; neither theory really made sense without the other. Galton needed stirp because stirp invalidated the inheritance of acquired characters. When Galton worried about the physiological basis of heredity, he was not participating in a scientific debate, he was actually having an argument with himself: "Can eugenics be given a scientific base?" Once we understand this we understand why he dropped the stirp theory so soon after proposing it; he was convinced of its validity and it really did not matter what others might think. Once he found a physiological explanation that made sense of his social theory, he dropped it—not realizing that perhaps he should have claimed it as a major contribution to the development of biology.

Galton's Contribution to Genetics and Biostatistics

Francis Galton was neither a proficient mathematician nor a skilled biologist, yet his work lies at the foundation of two of the most fruitful sciences of the twentieth century: biostatistics and genetics. He was not the first to apply probability laws to human populations (Quételet and Gould among others had done so earlier[149]) but until Galton's time biostatistics simply did not exist as a discipline unto itself. He provided the basic discoveries, the theoretical framework and the financial support that were needed to establish a full-fledged science. Others helped, Karl Pearson and W. F. R. Weldon to name just two, but it was Galton who galvanized their interest. In the early days of biostatistics he was the inspiration, the principal investigator, and the funding agency rolled into one.

Galton's work was also an inspiration for the men who founded genetics, although the reasons for this are more difficult to discern. His Ancestral Law of Heredity (that each parent contributes one-quarter of the heritage of an offspring, each grandparent one-eighth, etc) was rather quickly superseded by the rediscovery of Mendel's laws, these being more carefully derived, more useful, and considerably more generalizable. Galton was not the first to develop a particulate model of inheritance; Spencer and Darwin and many others had preceded him on that score, and, in any event, his stirp theory of inheritance never commanded much attention from biologists. Aside from his discovery of regression to the population mean there is no other datum of genetic knowledge that Galton can be said to have contributed. It remains true, nonetheless, that at least three of the men who created Mendelian genetics after 1900 (Bateson, deVries, and Johannsen) consciously based their work on a foundation that they believed Galton had laid. Subsequent historians of genetics, despite some difficulty in ascertaining precisely what it was that Galton did, have continued to assert that his contribution was significant.[150]

Thus we are confronted with something of a puzzle with regard to Galton, a puzzle that has two separate but equally perplexing parts. The first is, how could a rather naïve mathematician manage to discover two of the most powerful tools of statistical analysis? Second, how could that same person, a rather naïve biologist, not improperly be regarded as one of the founders of genetics?

The first of these puzzles can be solved by quickly retracing the path that led Galton to the discovery of regression and correlation. This account does an injustice to the historical record by leaving out the mistakes that he made and the conceptual deadends that he pursued along the way. For the moment, however, such an account is necessary in order to clarify an otherwise confusing picture.[151]

The trail originates in the pages of *Hereditary Genius* (1869) where Galton first used probability techniques to find a way of ranking intelligence and to estimate the number of men in Great Britain who would fall into each rank if a normal distribution of intelligence was assumed.[152] He was unable to compare his estimates with reality (that is, to test whether or not intelligence or any other characteristic of human populations were normally distributed) as he lacked a body of data, and in the years after 1869 he devoted a good part of his time to repairing that deficiency.

At first he thought about establishing a national registry in which the physical and mental attributes of the population could be recorded. Not long after he realized that a random sample of the population would suffice and also that children attending public schools could be one such sample if the officials in the schools would cooperate in measuring them.[153] The schools in fact did cooperate and Galton used the data on the height and weight of the students to investigate a question that he regarded as an important aspect of the eugenic program: whether children reared in the cities were physically less able than their counterparts in the countryside.[154] Having completed this analysis (of course he concluded that the answer was "yes") Galton realized that he needed data from at least two generations (fathers and sons) in order to determine whether the differences were hereditary. As he could not think of a likely and quick way to obtain data regarding the fathers of the public school boys he resolved to do an experiment on a population that would be easier to manipulate and quicker to reproduce. Ironically, the material that he chose was sweet-peas, but, unlike Mendel, he was asking specifically eugenic questions in his experiments: "It was anthropological evidence that I desired, caring only for the seeds as means of throwing light on heredity in Man."[155]

Galton sent sets of seed (seven bags, containing ten seeds each, all ten of the same diameter) to friends throughout the country (he did not have a garden at his home in London) and asked that the seeds be planted in seven rows and that the produce of each row be returned to him in the bags that had contained the parental seeds for the row. He wanted to find out whether the offspring of extreme parents (very small or very large seeds) would be as extreme as their parents, a precise analogue of finding out whether skinny fathers will have skinny sons. Seven of the experimental crops succeeded and in the winter of 1875–76 Galton had data from the produce of 490 seeds to analyze. As part of this analysis he decided to plot the diameter of the mother seeds against the diameter of the filial seeds; he marked the body of a graph wherever parental size and mean filial size intersected. When the marks were connected and some irregularities smoothed over he had drawn a straight line with a measurable slope. In modern terminology the first regression line had been drawn and the first regression coefficient had been measured.[156]

Galton did not at first understand the implications of what he had done; that graph, which with hindsight seems such a remarkable achievement, was not even used in the published version of the paper. The fact that offspring of extreme parents were closer to the population mean than their parents had been, seemed to him to be a natural concommitant of the fact (a fact whose truth he simply presumed) that the carriers of heredity were particulate and the processes of heredity probabilistic—and it was this aspect of his work that he chose to illustrate (see Fig. 2). The regression coefficient that he had calculated he termed a "reversion coefficient," as he thought it demonstrated why extreme members of a population tend to "revert" to type.

Within a decade after 1877 Galton came to realize that his coefficient of reversion was as much a product of his statistical manipulation as it was a product of hereditary phenomena, and he changed the name from "reversion" to "regression." During that decade he set himself to acquiring information on human populations, and to that end he established and managed an anthropometric laboratory at the South Kensington Health Exposition (and later at the South Kensington Science Museum), where individuals and families could have their vital measurements taken for a price. By 1885 he had acquired data on the vital statistics of 928 offspring and their parents. In the process of plotting and manipulating that data Galton discovered that reversion lines could be constructed whenever two populations were compared with each other—whether or not the two populations were genetically related. Plots of grouped data, plots which set individual offspring height against mean parental height, plots of frequencies and degrees of variation against each other, all produced reversion lines—and so the name had to be changed to something which did not necessarily imply hereditary connection.[157]

Galton had a gift for the visual representation of data. As a result of his continuing interest in meteorology and his association with the instrument-testing activities of Kew Observatory he also had had experience, prior to beginning his heredity work, with the plotting of large amounts of data on graphs. He did not possess, on the other hand, great facility with mathematics and often had to consult with others more expert in that domain to carry through the mathematical implications of some of his discoveries.[158] Thus the basis for his discovery of regression and correlation was fundamentally empir-

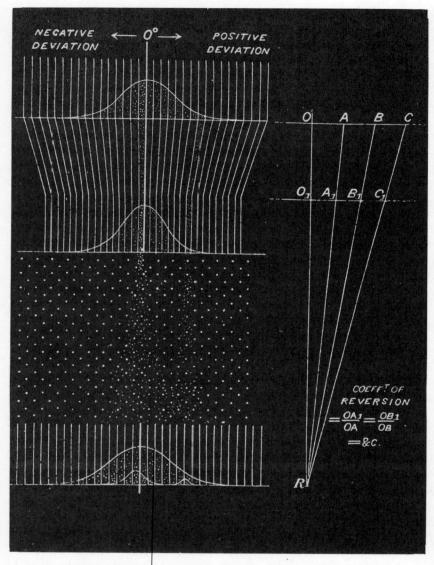

Fig. 2. Galton's model of reversion, as taken from *LLL* 2:9. The original appeared in *Typical laws of heredity,* Proceedings of the Royal Institution, Feb. 9, 1877.

ical and graphic rather than deductive and abstract. This is made particularly clear by Galton's own recollection of how he came to see the larger implications of regression analysis. In the process of charting the data that he had accumulated at the anthropometric laboratories he drew up a particularly meticulous graph in which the stature of every offspring was entered opposite that of its mid-parent (a weighted average of the two parental heights). In an effort to simplify the chart he decided to count the number of entries in each square inch of the table and the results were entered at the intersections of the appropriate horizontal and vertical lines (see Fig. 3).

I found it hard at first to catch the full significance of the entries, though I soon discovered curious and apparently very interesting relations between them. . . . Lines drawn through entries of the same value formed a series of concentric and similar ellipses. The common centre lay at the intersection of those vertical and horizontal lines which correspond to the value of 68½ inches [the population mean for both offspring and parents]. . . . Their axes were similarly inclined. The points where each successive ellipse was touched by a horizontal tangent, lay in a straight line that was inclined to the vertical in the ratio of ⅔ and those where the ellipses were touched by a vertical tangent, lay in a straight line inclined to the horizontal in the ratio ⅓.[159]

Galton also realized that the elliptical diagram could have been constructed using only three pieces of information: (1) the probable error for the parental generation; (2) the probable error for the filial generation; and (3) the average regression of the latter on the former. Mathematically it should have been possible to redraw his chart using nothing but those three pieces of information and the formulae for the conic sections. This, however, Galton could not himself do. He sent the problem out for solution to J. D. Hamilton Dickson, then tutor at St. Peter's College, Cambridge. "I wrote down these [three] values, and phrasing the problem in abstract terms, disentangled from all reference to heredity . . . I asked him kindly to investigate for me the Surface of Frequency of Error that would result from these three data, and the various shapes and other particulars of its sections that were made by horizontal planes."[160] Dickson's diagram was almost identical to the one that Galton had constructed. Dickson had confirmed deductively the conclusions that Galton had reached empirically. "I may be permitted to say that I never felt such a glow of loyalty and respect towards the sovereignty and magnificent sway of mathematical analysis as when his answer reached me confirming, by purely mathematical reasoning, my various and laborious statistical conclusions with far more minuteness than I had dared to hope, for the original data ran somewhat roughly, and I had to smooth them with tender caution."[161]

Although Galton referred to his charts of anthropometric data as "tables of co-relation" he still had not come to the discovery of correlation. This occurred a few years later as a result of his investigation of the system of personal identification pioneered by the French prison official Alphonse Ber-

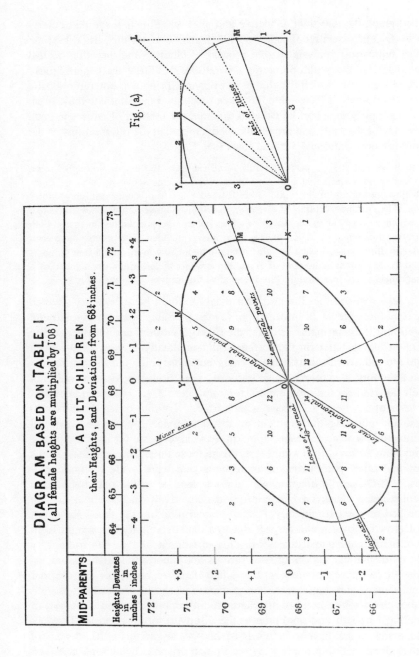

Fig. 3. Galton's elliptic contour, drawn from his observations, as reproduced in *LLL* 3:14.

tillon. Galton had been interested in personal identification for many years because he was searching for accurate measurements of resemblance between members of the same family. Bertillon had suggested that a unique profile could be developed for individuals (specifically, prisoners) by combining measurements of the head and limbs. After some months of musing over Bertillon's system Galton concluded that it would be more likely to produce type profiles than individual profiles because the measurements would not be independent variables; head breadth would be dependent upon head length and foot length would be dependent on toe length, etc.

Galton discovered correlation in trying to determine just how fallacious Bertillon's system might be. He constructed charts on which he plotted, for example, the arm length of individuals against their stature.

Not only did it turn out that the measure of correlation between two variables is exceedingly simple and definite, but it became evident almost from the first that I had unconsciously explored the very same ground before. No sooner did I begin to tabulate the data than I saw that they ran in just the same form as those that referred to family likeness in stature. . . . A very little reflection made it clear that family likeness was nothing more than a particular case of the wide subject of correlation, and that the whole of the reasoning already bestowed upon the special case of family likeness was equally applicable to correlation in its most general aspect.[162]

Thus Galton came to realize that regression coefficients can be derived even when the entities being compared are not "populations" and even when the measurements being compared are not commensurable. Lung capacity, for example, could be correlated with chest breadth as long as the two measurements were expressed in statistical units, degrees of deviation, and not in absolute units.

Thus for Galton the discovery of correlation was essentially the discovery that regression analysis was more generalizable than he had previously thought. Empirical investigation led him along this path, not mathematical intuition. Galton's flair for visual representation of data lies at the heart of his ability to discover these techniques, not his success at abstract reasoning. It was the charts that he created that signaled his breakthrough, not the mathematical analysis that subsequently made sense of them. This is the reason why, despite his ineptness as a mathematician, he was able to make two such fundamental mathematical discoveries.

That Galton was driven to proceed down this tortuous path from the rudimentary statistical techniques that he used in *Hereditary Genius* in 1869 to the more creative techniques that he discussed in *Natural Inheritance* twenty years later is a tribute to his commitment to the eugenic ideal and his compulsion to mathematize everything he studied. Before 1865 he had appeared, to himself and to others, to be something of a dilettante. After 1865 he was as a man transformed; the eugenic dream had transformed him and kept him at his work. All of the investigations that he pursued with enthusiasm (the studies of biographical dictionaries, the pangenesis experiments, the school statistics, the anthropometric statistics, Bertillon's system of personal identification) were motivated by his desire to provide an objective foundation upon which to build the perfect eugenic state. All of these experiments and investigations (except the series on pangenesis) were mathematical at a time when quantification was most unusual in anthropology and in the nonphysiological areas of biology. All of his theories and models were visual in delivery and impact. All of his statistical ideas were generated out of empirical study rather than reached by means of deductive reasoning.

Galton's fierce determination to pursue the facts of heredity and to pursue them mathematically also lies at the root of his contribution to genetics.[163] For at the most rudimentary level (and that is the level at which Galton was working) in order to study something mathematically you have to be able to count it, and in order to count it you must have a fairly clear definition of what it is. In addition, if you want to make your study scientific, a definition must be shared by at least a few other people. It is no use trying to find a way to demarcate different kinds of mice on the basis of body length if one group of taxonomists measures their mice alive, another group measures theirs skinned, a third includes the length of the whiskers in the overall measurements, and a fourth excludes the length of the tails. There must be some mutual agreement about the limits of the phenomenon to be studied.

This is precisely what had not happened in heredity studies at the time that Galton began his work. Before 1869 the word "heredity" was barely used in scientific discourse and the phenomena that it might demarcate were undefined. "The current views on Heredity were at that time so vague and contradictory that it is difficult to summarize them briefly. . . . It seems hardly credible now that even the word heredity was then considered fanciful and unusual. I was chaffed by a cultured friend for adopting it from the French."[164] The word "inheritance" was occasionally used (for example, Darwin called the theory of pangenesis a theory of inheritance), but the unacknowledged trouble with "inheritance" lay in the fact that it had a variety of definitions, depending upon the context in which it was being used.

The usual formulation was to call "inheritance" the "tendency for like to reproduce like," but between that statement and a rigorous understanding of what it meant there was a wide gap indeed. Inheritance was, for example, often confused with "reversion," the tendency for ancestral characteristics to reassert themselves after having been lost for one or several generations. Sometimes inheritance and reversion were discussed as if they were opposites: the tendency of parents to assert their characteristics in opposition to the tendency of more remote ancestors to assert theirs. Other times inheritance and reversion were discussed as if the latter were a special case of the former:

the tendency of some ancestral characteristics to be so strong that they dominate over other, newer characteristics. In the first form of defining the difference between inheritance and reversion the two opposing forces are carried by individuals (parents and more remote ancestors). In the second form of definition the two complementary forces are carried by traits (such as whiteness of feathers in pigeons or blueness of eyes in humans).

If the distinction between inheritance and reversion was murky, it nonetheless was in no way so obscure as the distinction between variation and inheritance. Sometimes inheritance was said to be the tendency for like to reproduce like and variation was said to be an opposing force, causing like to reproduce unlike, or causing children to be slightly different from their parents. Of course, it was by no means clear where inheritance ended and variation began when making measurements of actual organisms; whether, for example, a 6¼″ tail in the offspring of parents with a 6½″ tail was to be regarded as a product of natural perturbations in inheritance or a product of an opposing force leading to variation. In other contexts variation was discussed as if it were a form of reversion (ancestors reasserting themselves), or sometimes as a product of environmental influences asserted upon the hereditary constitution.[165]

The debate about the nature of variation had been going on for several years before 1859. After the publication of the *Origin of Species,* however, it became even more heated (and confused) because inheritance, reversion and variation were crucial concepts in the theory of evolution by natural selection. Among other confusing questions was the issue of whether there was a real distinction between individual (small) variations and discontinuous (large) ones—and whether one or the other was to be considered evolutionarily significant.

Thus when Galton began his study of heredity in 1865 there was no common agreement amongst biologists about the definitions of the phenomena to be studied, and the phenomena themselves, ill-defined as they were, were embroiled in one of the most emotional scientific debates of all time. That Galton was essentially untutored in biology must have been a blessing in disguise. He was not a participant in the debate about inheritance and he was not really involved in the debate about evolution by natural selection—both of which he simply accepted as given. From the start he was convinced that *everything* was hereditary (the eugenicist's fundamental tenet) and was therefore never plagued with doubts about whether reversion and variation were really part of the picture. Since individuals did in fact vary from their parents, and since long lost characters did in fact reassert themselves, variation and reversion could not be denied. Since, however, *everything* was heredity (note, not inheritance), variation and reversion had to be subsumed under that larger head.

Galton's notion that heredity was probabilistic was the key; both reversion and variation could be subsumed under heredity if heredity were particulate and if there were such a large number of particles that their behavior could be described probabilistically. Both Galton's Law of Ancestral Heredity and his discovery of regression to the population mean implied that infinitely distant ancestors contribute to the heritage of each offspring. In this way reversion could be understood as a chance result of the processes of generation. The same was true of individual small variations, which Galton could show to be nothing more nor less than the probabilistic concommitant of particulate inheritance, nothing more nor less than the random distribution of independent characters.[166]

One of the consequences of this probabilistic analysis of individual variation was the realization that since chance processes are always operating, individual variations will be normally distributed from generation to generation. Thus individual variation would act to preserve a species type rather than to destroy it. If individual small variations were not the material from which our natural selection was to work, then discontinuous large variations had to be. It was the large variations, the jumps, the "mutations" as deVries came to call them, which provided grist for the mill of evolution. This was one aspect of Galton's work that his contemporaries, particularly William Bateson, found particularly stimulating.[167]

Yet, on the basis of this analysis, we can see that Galton's contribution to genetics actually goes much deeper than his understanding of the importance of discontinuous variation, as significant as that may be. Basically, what Galton did was to define the territory that genetics could explore by collapsing three entities—inheritance, variation, and reversion—into one—heredity. He then went one step further, a step that was required by his desire to make the study of heredity mathematical. If every attribute that an individual possessed was possessed by virtue of heredity then the force of heredity could be measured in the outward appearance of the individual or individuals. Resemblance between individuals was the crucial indicator. There was, truth to tell, nothing else that a student of heredity *could* have counted in the days before the discovery that chromosomes carried the hereditary material, but Galton made virtue out of necessity. By measuring heredity in the outward appearance of individuals he defined heredity as the relationship (and difference) between individuals, and it was on this definition and its attendant assumptions that the new science of genetics was built.

Contemporaries of Galton's understood that this was the case. J. A. Thomson aptly summarized the change in the meaning of heredity that Galton had effected: "By heredity we do not mean the general fact of observation that like tends to beget like, nor a power making for continuity or persistence of characters—to be opposed to the power of varying—nor anything but *the organic or genetic relation between successive* generations: and by "inheritance" we mean "organic inheritance": *all that the organism is or has to start with in virtue of its hereditary relation to parents and ancestors.*"[168] William Bateson commented that heredity studies had been saved from disorder by Galton's emphasis on studying the "outward facts of transmission. We do not know," he continued,

what is the essential agent in the transmission of parental characters, not even whether it is a material agent or not. Not only is our ignorance complete, but no one has the remotest idea how to set to work on that part of the problem. . . .
But . . . we can study the outward facts of transmission. Here, if our knowledge is still very vague, we are at least beginning to see how we ought to go to work. . . . [I]t has become likely that general expressions will be found capable of sufficiently wide application to be justly called "laws" of heredity. That this is so, is due almost entirely to the work of Mr. F. Galton.[169]

Galton's concept of heredity—incorporating inheritance, reversion, and variation and measurable in the physical appearance of populations—was also inseparable from his eugenic ideal and from his early passion for counting. It was the eugenic ideal that led him to the conviction that everything was hereditary, and it was his passion for counting that led him to search for something to measure and for probabilistic models. Ironically, the spread of this definition among literate men was also dependent upon the eugenic ideal, because it was through the growth and development of the eugenics movement that the definition became part of the intellectual currency of a new generation.

Galton Last Years

The last decades of Francis Galton's life must have been a time of great satisfaction for him, despite the loss of family and friends and despite the gradual erosion of his health. Between 1890 and 1911 he witnessed the success of much of what he had believed in and fought for earlier in his life. Those who knew him well during those years remarked that he never acquired that certain pessimism, that despair of the future, that longing for past pleasantries that often characterize the aged and the infirm. Until his death Francis Galton remained an optimist, with the curiosity and the freshness of spirit of a much younger man.[170]

And with good reason. In the last decade of his life the eugenic state that he had first conceived in the 1860s, looked as if it might—slowly—become reality. Politicians began to ask him and his disciples for advice. The number of his disciples grew. The doctrine spread to other lands, to America and to

Germany especially. "Eugenics" became part of the English language. All this Galton lived to see and to delight in.

Similarly, between 1890 and 1911 his scientific work began at last to bear fruit. Earlier in his life he had been alone in his work. In England there were few scientists who could understand and appreciate what he was about. After 1889, after *Natural Inheritance,* this situation changed. Galton found himself at the head of a school, master to his disciples, benefactor of institutes and laboratories to carry on his work, winner of honorary medals, honorary fellow of Trinity College, widely acclaimed and widely heralded as the founder of a new science—biostatistics—and widely praised for having understood the significance of a new biological principle—heredity—earlier than anyone else.

What had changed? Was it Francis Galton, or was it the world around him that had been transformed? Had Galton, by virtue of his years of contact with biological professionals, finally matured to the point of understanding the questions, the principles, and the methods that were important to them? Or had the biological profession, by virtue of the accretion of new knowledge and the insufficiency of old theories, finally come to need the kind of insight that Galton was prepared to provide? Similarly, what had happened in the political sphere? Had Galton finally found a way to present eugenics in a politically attractive fashion? Or had England (and America) by virtue of decades of unfulfilled flirtation with the democratic egalitarian ideal, finally become ready to accept a steadying dose of old fashioned fatalistic elitism?

In both spheres—the political and the biological—all the available evidence points to the same conclusion: Francis Galton had not changed substantially. After 1889 Galton did not become more attuned to the concerns of traditional biologists; if anything, as his own methodology acquired adherents he and his disciples became less capable of joining the mainstream of the biological community, at the very same time that that stream began flowing closer to his own. Similarly, eugenics as Galton presented it after 1889 was hardly a diluted, moderated version of the eugenics he had first suggested in 1865. If anything, his views had hardened, become more rigid and more forthright—but England had changed so thoroughly in the intervening decades that what had seemed odd, if not a bit offensive (marriages made for the good of the state? breed people as we breed horses?) in 1870 began to appear reasonable and attractive by 1910. The last decades of Galton's life overlapped the last years of Victoria's reign and the advent of her son, Edward—the "strange death of liberal England." Galton discovered, in the last years of his life, that his time had finally come.

The range of Francis Galton's interests did not narrow in his declining years; if anything, it became broader. Meteorology remained a passion. The anthropometric researches that had absorbed so much of his time in the 1880s were replaced by researches on fingerprints. As avidly as he had once collected data about height, weight, and eye color, he now collected prints from members of different races and families. The problem of measuring the physical resemblance between individuals continued to fascinate him; in 1901 he experimented with a technique for panoramic photography, so that the whole of a face could be represented in one snapshot. As late as 1906 he wrote a memoir on the subject of physical resemblance (unpublished), suggesting a way to measure the critical distance at which a face is just barely recognizable. Between 1889 and 1911 he traveled extensively, just as he had in the past. In the winter of 1899 he undertook what must have been an exhausting trip to Egypt, to which he had not returned since the adventurous days of his youth. "Today we had an excursion of seven hours, including about 14 miles of donkey ride. I was lucky in beast and saddle and enjoyed it as much as any horse ride that I can recollect. The wonders are just unspeakable."[171] Through all these years he kept up a lively correspondence with members of his family, with friends, and with the growing crowd of biometricians. His administrative work at the Royal Society and the British Association declined during these years, owing in part to his advancing deafness. He filled the void with the problems of organizing a new journal, *Biometrika,* and financing the Eugenics Laboratory at University College, London. Aside from his writings on biometry, eugenics, and fingerprints, he published short papers on such varied subjects as a cure for gout, the number of strokes of a brush in a picture, cutting a round cake on scientific principles, improving the literary style of scientific papers, and sequestrated church property.[172] Through it all Galton never outgrew his passion for counting and measuring, a particularly telling example of which occurs in a letter to his niece in 1905: "I have had a stern reminder not to delay, in the form of a sudden severe shivering for nearly a couple of hours on Wednesday morning. The *amplitude* of the shiver was remarkable and interesting; my hands shook through a range of fully 7 if not 8 inches.[173] His physical powers declined as the years wore on, but his intellectual prowess never diminished. He was as interested in the world around him in his eighty-fifth year as he had been in his forty-fifth, if anything about that world particularly fascinated him it was the possibility of counting and measuring it.

And changing it. To the end Galton never relinquished his passionate desire to improve the world. Eugenics, and Galton's hopes for it, had been the crucial factor that transformed him from a youthful dilettante into a mature and disciplined investigator. Eugenics had carried him through the arduous years of work on anthropometric statistics and theorizing about heredity. Now, eugenics became even more important; it dominated his life. "I live quite as much in Kantsawa [an early spelling of Kantsaywhere, his eugenic Utopia] as I do in Haslemere,[174] he wrote to his niece in 1910, and, speaking figuratively, he was not exaggerating.

Galton's fingerprint studies illustrate this eugenic compulsion. He was interested in fingerprints because he was interested in personal identification, which interested him because he hoped that he could use degrees of resemblance to measure the strength of heredity. "It has long been my hope," he had written in 1888, "though utterly without direct experimental corroboration thus far, that if a considerable number of variables and independent features could be catalogued it might be possible to trace kinship with considerable certainty.[175] After 1888 Galton pursued fingerprints earnestly.

He took prints of his family, his friends, his acquaintances, and 2,500 persons who visited his anthropometric laboratory. By 1891 he had satisified himself that the prints were unique to each individual, that they possessed regularities which permitted classification, and that they persisted unaltered through the life of the individual and by 1892 he had published a book on the subject.[176] The next year a Parliamentary Committee recommended, after extensive visits to Galton's laboratory, that fingerprinting be adopted as the sole method for identifying criminals in England.[177]

But Galton was not satisfied; he wanted to know something more. He wanted to prove that the ridge patterns were hereditary, passed from generation to generation and distinctive for each race.[178] Throughout his life, as we have seen, Galton practiced the art of differential skepticism. Though he could be acutely critical of methodological and logical faults in someone else's work, he was equally capable of throwing caution to the winds when he was in pursuit of a point that he desperately wanted to make. So it was with the inheritance of fingerprints. By dividing prints into three separate types (Arch, Loop, Whorl) and by comparing the prints of 105 pairs of siblings, he found that the number of siblings that had prints of the same type was slightly higher than the number to be expected by chance (e.g., there were 42 cases of both siblings with loop patterns; chance predicted 37.6); Galton concluded that the patterns must be hereditary. This procedure was somewhat dubious. The sample was small, the classifications probably inappropriate, and the statistical procedure questionable.[179] Yet he was determined to see inheritance, so inheritance was precisely what he saw. The same thing happened in his analysis of race. Though he could not find a distinctive pattern for the English, Welsh, Hebrew, and Negro races (the only ones for which he had data), he did find that the percentage of arches in the prints of each race varied from 7.9 for Jews to 13.6 for the English. The samples of English, Welsh, and Negroes were too small to allow a significant conclusion (the differences could be due to random error) yet Galton remarked, "Still, whether it be from pure fancy on my part, or from some real peculiarity, the general aspect of the Negro print strikes me as characteristic. . . . [T]hey give an idea of greater simplicity, due to causes that I have not yet succeeded in submitting to the test of measurement."[180]

Galton did not take the problem of inheritance in fingerprint patterns any farther than this, but the episode serves to illustrate that in the last two decades of his life his fundamental scientific goal had not changed. Despite all that he had learned of statistics and evolution in the interim, he was just as intent to prove the omnicompetence of heredity in 1893 as he had been in 1865, at whatever methodological cost. He began his scientific career convinced that nature dominated over nurture, and thirty years later his conviction had not waned. If anything, it was stronger.

Just as his prime motive for scientific work did not change in the last decades of his life, so too his major biological ideas, codified in *Natural Inheritance,* remained unaltered in succeeding years. The rediscovery of Mendel's papers in 1901—papers which he should have been uniquely qualified to appreciate, given his passion for statistics in biology—was an event of almost no significance for him.[181] Perhaps, by 1901, he was too old to absorb the new ideas. Perhaps he was simply too involved in eugenic matters to pay much attention to new developments in biological theory. There is some evidence that indicates that Galton's attitude toward Mendelism was favorable, although never enthusiastic. In the autumn of 1904 Galton wrote several letters to William Bateson in which he suggested his willingness to accept Mendelism. He even expressed a hope that some of his own investigations would prove to be of theoretical value for the Mendelians.[182]

Nothing in Galton's set of biological ideas necessarily mitigated against his ability to understand and appreciate the significance of Mendel's work, despite his lack of enthusiasm. In the first place, he believed that discontinuous variation was the basis for evolutionary change, one of the cardinal tenets of Mendelism. In his publications after 1889 he frequently reiterated his stand on this issue.[183] "I have frequently insisted that these sports or 'aberrances' (if I may coin the word) are probably notable factors in the evolution of races. Certainly the successive improvements of breeds of domestic animals generally . . . make fresh starts from decided sports or aberrances, and are by no means always developed slowly through the accumulation of minute and favourable variations during a long succession of generations."[184]

Galton believed in discontinuous variation at a time when that belief was itself aberrant. He had two reasons for doing so: one was biological, the other typically eugenic. On biological grounds it was clear to him that the law of regression, which said that the offspring of deviate parents will be less deviate than their parents, implied a deep conservatism in nature. Regression kept the characteristics of a population intact; and kept them from spreading too far from type. Since regression was a concomittant of normal variation, normal variation could not produce new types, another mechanism was necessary—the sport, the aberrance, or, as we would say, the mutation. Only a sport could, according to Galton, make the individual so deviate that his or her offspring would fail to regress toward the old racial type.

Galton's eugenic rationale for discontinuous variation was particularly interesting. If evolution proceeded by imperceptible steps, he reasoned, the improvement of the human race would take forever, or at least a very long time, longer than the life of any man now alive. If evolution proceeded by sports, however, that time would be drastically shortened. Dramatic changes could be seen in one or two generations. Francis Galton was always an optimist; forever was too long for him to wait.

Inquiries are greatly needed into the discontinuous variations of human faculty. . . . The assurance that sports of considerable magnitude occasionally occur in moral and intellectual gifts, justifies more daring speculations than we are apt to indulge, in respect both to the past and future history of mankind. It does not seem to me by any means so certain as is commonly supposed by the scienfific men of the present time, that our evolution from a brute ancestry was through a series of severally imperceptible advances. Neither does it seem by any means certain that humanity must linger for an extremely long time at or about its present unsatisfactory level. As a matter of fact, the Greek race of the classical times have surpassed in natural faculty all other races before or since, and some future race may be at least the equal of the Greek, while it is reasonable to hope that when the power of heredity and the importance of preserving valuable ''transiliencies'' [sports] shall have become generally recognised, effective efforts will be made to preserve them.[185]

Galton's principal disciples, Karl Pearson and W. F. R. Weldon, adamantly opposed discontinuous variation as the basis for evolutionary change, and this contention was one of the factors in their bitter dispute with the Mendelians.[186] Galton was not a neutral bystander to that dispute, but it is worth noting that on this crucial point he did not entirely agree with his own disciples.

Nonetheless, despite Galton's belief in discontinuous variation he remained more or less impervious to the rediscovery of Mendel's Laws. He seemed not to have noticed that anything of special significance had happened in heredity studies after 1901. Galton was fond of his Ancestral Law, and it was indeed different from Mendel's Laws. This, combined with his age, his involvement with eugenics, and his fondness for the biometricians who were battling the Mendelians, may well have kept him from expressing more interest in Mendelism than he did. Consequently, in the last decade of his life, when his favorite branch of science, the study of heredity, was undergoing an upheaval that would transform it completely, Galton's ideas about heredity remained unchanged.

This helps us to understand an apparent paradox in Galton's life. For years he had advocated quantitative studies of hereditary phenomena and had insisted that evolution proceeded by big jumps and not by small variations. Yet just at the time when the general biological community began, finally, to agree with him, he found himself in the opposition camp. That situation was not really of his own making, but was due in large part to the fractious personalities of William Bateson and Karl Pearson.

Until the publication of *Natural Inheritance* Galton had been a scientific loner; very few "men of note" had expressed more than passing interest in his work. Not long after the book appeared he made his first convert: W. F. R. Weldon was a marine biologist of the classical sort. A young man (he was born the year after the publication of the *Origin of Species*), he had been trained at Cambridge and had, in 1890, become Jodrell professor of zoology at University College, London.[187] Weldon was smitten with Galton's statistical method and proposed to do several studies of variation in the shrimp, *Crangon vulgaris*.[188] In 1891 Weldon began to learn probability theory and sought the help of his colleague at University College, Karl Pearson.[189] Pearson, three years Weldon's senior, was professor of applied mathematics and mechanics. He had had a passing interest in statistics, largely as it pertained to problems in the philosophy of science, but Weldon's enthusiasm seems to have been contagious. Pearson very quickly became a devotee, assisting Weldon in his statistical work and, not long after, publishing studies of his own.

By the end of the decade Weldon and Pearson had constituted themselves as Galton's school. The three men wrote to each other, they visited socially, they spent vacations and holidays together, they trained students, founded laboratories, began a journal (about which more below), celebrated at "biometric teas," and even coined a private name for themselves, "the passionate statisticians."[190] It is scarcely surprising that when Pearson and Weldon were attacked, Galton, no matter what his feelings on the validity of the attack, rallied to their support.

That the attack was mounted by William Bateson was a bitter irony; on the basis of their biological beliefs Galton and Bateson should have been colleagues, not enemies. Galton was one of the very few reviewers who gave favorable notice to Bateson's book, *Materials for the Study of Variation* (1894).[191] "I don't think many people admire, or can admire, Mr. Galton more than I do," wrote Bateson to Galton's grandniece in 1909, "How often have I regretted that Mr. Galton has not been with us in the past ten years. [Bateson is referring here to the battle between the Mendelians and the biometricians; Galton was still alive when the letter was written.] It has been indeed a strange perversity of chance."[192]

Almost a contemporary of Weldon and Pearson, and trained at Cambridge, as they had been, Bateson started his career with studies of invertebrate embryology, just as Weldon had; Weldon had, in fact, helped to stimulate Bateson's interest in the subject.[193] By the 1890s Bateson had shifted to studies of variation and had become convinced that discontinuous variation was the basis of evolutionary change. His monumental catalogue, *Materials for the Study of Variation,* was subtitled, appropriately, *Treated with Especial Regard to Discontinuity in the Origin of Species.*

The battle between Bateson and the biometricians was first joined on precisely this issue. In 1894, at Galton's urging, the Royal Society created a Committee for the Measurement of Plants and Animals. Its members included two young biologists, E. B. Poulton and A. M. Meldola, as well as Galton and Weldon. In 1895 the Committee published its first report, a paper by Weldon, "Attempt to Measure the Death Rate Due to Selective Destruction of *Carcinas moenas* with Respect to a Particular Dimension," to which was appended a more theoretical discussion, also by Weldon, "Remarks on Variation in Animals and Plants." Weldon argued that small, continuous variations were the most likely source of change in evolution.[194]

Bateson was furious and showered several critical letters upon Galton and the Committee.[195] In 1897, perhaps in an effort at compromise, Bateson was appointed to the Committee. Pearson had been appointed the year before, along with several zoologists and breeders who were not noticeably interested in measurement. The scope of the Committee was changed, as was its name; thenceforth it became the Evolution Committee of the Royal Society.

And thenceforth its troubles began. The gap between the statistically inclined members (Galton, Pearson, and Weldon) and the "older type" biologists (particularly Bateson) grew wider. The statisticians wished to support studies of large populations, the others insisted that only careful examination of individual cases would produce useful results. "I wanted to write a few words to you about yesterday's meeting," Pearson wrote Galton shortly after the Committee had been enlarged,

... I felt badly out of place in such a gathering of biologists, and little capable of expressing opinions which would only have hurt their feelings . . . I always succeed in creating hostility without getting others to see my views. . . .

I believe that your problems [a list Galton had composed of pressing problems in heredity and variation] could be answered by direct and well devised experiments . . . [b]ut I venture to think that the Committee you have got together is entirely unsuited to direct such experiments. It is far too large, contains far too many of the old biological type, and is far too unconscious of the fact that the solutions to these problems *are in the first place statistical, and in the second place statistical, and only in the third place biological* [italics mine].[196]

To this Galton replied, perhaps sensing what lay ahead, "It must always be borne in mind that we are dealing with human workers, who have their own ideas which must be respected and humoured, if we are to gain their cordial cooperation. We have, to speak rather grandly, *statesmanship* problems to deal with."[197]

But matters did not improve. The argument came to a head in 1900, when Pearson submitted a paper for publication by the Royal Society and it was sent to Bateson as one referee. Bateson submitted an unfavorable report. At the time the paper was read he appeared at the Royal Society meeting and denounced all of Pearson's work. Bateson's critical report was printed and distributed to the Fellows of the Royal Society before the paper was actually published in the *Philosophical Transactions* in November of the following year. Shortly after the acceptance of his paper Pearson received a note from the Council of the Society asking that he refrain from mixing statistics and biology in the future. Pearson considered resigning from the Royal Society, but finally resigned only from the Evolution Committee. Later in the year Galton and Weldon followed suit. In 1901 they founded *Biometrika*. Its first issue contained prefatory remarks by Galton in which he made it perfectly clear that the journal had been created because of the "coldness of welcome often afforded to a new departure in science."[198]

Thus, the antipathy between Bateson and the biometricians predated the rediscovery of Mendel's paper. Given their mutual dislike, it was a fair guess that any cause supported by Bateson would have been opposed by the biometricians, even if it were charities for widows and orphans. As it happened, the cause that Bateson adopted was Mendelism, and the fight between Bateson and biometricians became the battle between the Galtonians and the Mendelians.

The details of that battle do not concern us here so much as its results. Most of the biometricians were not biologists (except for Weldon) and most of the Mendelians were. The major biological and scientific journals did not carry papers by the biometricians because of the existence of *Biometrika;* consequently, most biologists did not read what they had to say. In any event, it was unlikely that the biologists would have understood the statistical arguments had they read them, as few biologists had mathematical training in those years.

Francis Galton found himself hoisted upon his own petard; he had advocated quantitative studies of heredity at a time when biologists were immersed in descriptive and taxonomic work. Just at the time when biologists began to change their point of departure, Galton became father to a school of statisticians who had long ago passed through the stage of counting to the stage of computing and who were now thinking in terms of correlation coefficients and standard deviations. Galton could hardly desert his own followers; consequently he found himself at odds with the biological community and isolated from the mainstream of biological thought.

In all likelihood this did not trouble him greatly because in the last decade of his life something of greater importance had happened to him. Isolated from the mainstream of biological thought, he was, nonetheless, swimming right(the pun is intended) with the tide of political thought, and that was, after all, what he most wished to be doing. Having dreamt his eugenic dream for so many years alone, he began to discover, after the turn of the century, that other men were willing to listen and to join him in his reverie.

The most important of these men was Karl Pearson, for it was Pearson who first encouraged Galton to articulate his eugenic ideas publicly, after so many years of keeping them to himself. Pearson was no stranger to the realms of political theory. In the 1880s he had been active in London socialist circles, had lectured on Marx, contributed to the *Socialist Songbook,* advocated women's rights, and published a relatively radical work of his own, *The Ethic of Free Thought.*[199] His political activity had diminished in the nineties, either because of the pressure of his statistical work, his growing family responsibilities, or his disillusionment with socialist theory. In any event, political concerns were never very far from the edge of his consciousness, and they surfaced again early in 1901.

Late in 1900 Pearson had delivered a lecture entitled "National Life from the Standpoint of Science" and sent Galton a copy.[200] "Thank you much for the 'Lecture.' It fits in with much that I habitually think about," Galton replied.[201] Apparently buoyed by Pearson's interest Galton went on to confide a scheme for awarding certificates of hereditary worth to young men who pass certain tests of physique, character, and intelligence.

... would then [the certificates] meet a want, and would they help in forwarding marriages of the fittest and discouraging others in any notable degree? If a well considered answer be "Yes" I suppose the action would be to write an article upon it . . . and then if the idea should *take,* to follow mainly the direction in which "the cat may jump."

I have thought over the subject a good deal and have more to say, but unless what *has* been said above seems reasonable to persons like yourself, the supplementary remarks would be useless. Will you kindly think this over at odd times during the next 2 or 3 days. I have written about it to no one else.[202]

Pearson was as enthusiastic as Galton had been hesitant. "It would be a very great pleasure to me to know you were going to take the field with regard to what I am convinced is of the greatest national importance—the breeding from the fitter stocks," he wrote to Galton just three days later.

If one could only get someone to awaken the nation with regard to its future! What . . . it seems to me we mostly need at the present time, is some word in season, something that will bring home to thinking men the urgency of the fertility question in this country. *There is no man who would be listened to in the same way as yourself* [italics mine].[203]

Galton was quick to answer Pearson's call. In the last week of January he departed for the Mediterranean and took with him a notebook that he filled with plans for a eugenic utopia, an experimental community, organized on the estate of the "Donoghues of Dunnoweir," for the purposes of inculcating eugenic ideals and facilitating the breeding of exceptionally fit individuals.[204] This scheme was still on his mind when he returned from his holiday. Somewhat later in the spring, when he was asked to be the Huxley Lecturer at the Royal Anthropological Society, he decided to devote his remarks to potential improvements of mankind.

"That [topic] which I have selected for tonight is one which has occupied my thoughts for many years and to which a large part of my published writings have borne a direct though silent reference," he began, and went on to describe the normal distribution of talent in human populations, the improvement that could be hoped for if only the highly talented were permitted to breed, ways to measure and award certificates for high talent, and ways to encourage higher birth rates among talented couples. The Donoghues of Dunnoweir appeared in a passing suggestion that great landowners who regularly employ and house young couples on their estates might "gather fine specimens of humanity around them, just as they gather fine breeds of cattle and horses." Galton ended, not atypically considering the time and place, with a short panegyric to the special glories and responsibilities of the White Man's Burden: "To no nation is a higher human breed more necessary than to our own for we plant our stock all over the world and lay the foundation of the dispositions and capacities of future millions of the human race."

In England the lecture seems to have fallen on deaf ears. The Anthropological Society never published it in full, and the columns of *Nature,* where it did appear, contained no subsequent letters or comments upon it. In America the reverse was true; the response was enthusiastic. Galton's lecture was published in the *Annual Report of the Smithsonian Institution,* and most crucially, in *Popular Science Monthly,* then one of the leading journals of scientific opinion in the United States.[205] "From America came an enormous amount of enthusiasm—letters of quasi-adoration such as *could* only hail from America."[206]

Thus encouraged Galton persevered and resolved, Pearson tells us, to appeal to the public and utilize the popular press in the future.[207] Accordingly, his next published statement on eugenics appeared in the *Daily Chronicle* in 1903.[208] Events began to conspire in his favor. Most crucially, the disasters of the Boer War had produced a mood of national self-doubt in Britain. By 1903 the appointment of a Royal Commission to study the deterioration of the English race was probably not as startling an event as it might have been had it happened ten years before.

The time was clearly ripe for Galton to act. In 1904 he gave £1500 to the University of London to establish a Research Fellowship in Eugenics and to support a Eugenics Record Office. In that year he also delivered a lecture, "Eugenics, Its Definition, Scope and Aims," to a large and enthusiastic audience, including H. G. Wells, Benjamin Kidd, George Bernard Shaw, L.

T. Hobhouse, and C. S. Lock.[209] In 1906, thanks to another grant from Galton, the Eugenics Record Office expanded to become the Francis Galton Eugenics Laboratory; Pearson was made director. A year later Galton gave the Herbert Spencer lecture at Oxford, again on eugenics.[210]

Galton's efforts began to bear fruit, and eugenic ideas started to percolate down to the general public. "You will be amused to know how general now is the use of your word *Eugenics*!" Pearson wrote to Galton, "I hear most respectable middle-class matrons saying, if children are weakly, 'Ah that was not a eugenic marriage!' "[211] In an effort to increase the downward flow of eugenic ideas, the Eugenic Education Society was founded in 1908 and soon began publishing a journal, *Eugenics Review*.[212]

The subsequent history of the eugenics movement need not detain us here. Enough has been said to indicate that what had been a very private and personal dream of Galton's as far back as 1865 had become, by the time of his death in 1911, a matter of public policy. For almost forty years Galton had hesitated to bring his dream into the light of day, confident, as he was, that the public reaction would be negative. In 1901 that hesitancy disappeared, and Galton began to realize that his eugenic ideas were touching a responsive chord in the English-speaking public.

Why was that chord responsive? The answer is not difficult to find. For various reasons there was a groundswell of antidemocratic, antiegalitarian, antienvironmentalist, elitist opinion in Britain and the United States in the first decade of the twentieth century.[213] Thoughtful contemporaries were aware of what was happening: "The great political revolution which began one hundred years ago . . . has well-nigh attained its ends . . . We have in reality entered on a new stage of social evolution in which the minds of men are moving towards other goals; and those political parties which still stand confronting the people with remnants of the political programme of political equality are beginning to find that the world is rapidly moving beyond their standpoint."[214]

Having enacted into law so many of the ideas of Bentham, Smith, and Mill, the British people were grieved to discover that the great millenium had not come to pass; "the greatest good for the greatest number," had produced some monumental changes in the British social and political systems, but it had failed to eliminate poverty, misery, revolutionary sentiment, and other social ills. If anything, those ills appeared to be aggravated, not improved.

Eugenics was the perfect political program to capitalize on this resurgence of conservative opinion. Grounded in biological theory, not physical theory as political economy had been, it was perfectly suited to the metaphors of the post-Darwinian age. Antiegalitarian in the extreme, it was the perfect counterweight to decades of democratic sentiment.

An average man is morally and intellectually an uninteresting being. The class to which he belongs is bulky and no doubt serves to help the course of social life in action. . . . But the average man is of no direct help towards evolution, which appears to . . . be the goal of all living existence. . . .

Some thoroughgoing democrats may look with complacency on a mob of mediocrities, but to most other persons they are the reverse of attractive. . . . All men would find themselves at nearly the same dead average level, each being as heavily endowed as his neighbor.[215]

Eugenic doctrine was antiurban at a time when fear of the cities was becoming rampant. It was racist at a time when the conflicts between the races were becoming everywhere apparent, in the United States and in the British Empire, at home and abroad. Most significantly, eugenic doctrine congratulated Anglo-Saxons on the superiority of their civilization at a time when they were beginning to feel insecure about their role in the world. Francis Galton had good reason to remain optimistic and enthusiastic in the last decades of his life. His eugenic dream appeared to be coming true. His family and friends must have been very grateful that he did not live to see what happened next.

NOTES

1. A vast collection of primary materials relating to Galton's life has been assembled in the library of University College, London; this collection, which was not catalogued at the time that I consulted it, will be referred to hereafter as *GA* (Galton Archive). An index catalogue for the archive has subsequently been prepared by the staff of the library but it arrived on my desk after this article had already been set in type. Many of the crucial materials in the archive were published in Karl Pearson, *Life, Letters and Labours of Francis Galton*, 4 vols. (Cambridge, 1914–30), which will be cited hereafter as *LLL*.

2. *Hereditary talent and character*, Macmillan's Magazine 12 (June 1865): 157–66; 12 (August 1965): 318–27.

3. *Hereditary talent and character*, p. 157. For the sake of simplicity page references to this article will appear subsequently in the body of the text.

4. Many of these objections were raised by Galton's contemporaries, especially after his theories were published in expanded form in *Hereditary Genius* (London, 1869). For example, Alphonse de Candolle, *Histoire des sciences et des savants depuis deux siècles* (Genève, 1873), and [Herman Merivale], *Hereditary genius*, Edinburgh Review 132 (July 1870): 100–25. Galton discussed some of the difficulties in his original argument in the introduction to the second edition of *Hereditary Genius* (London, 1892).

5. Marc J. Haller, *Eugenics, Hereditarian Attitudes in American Thought* (New Brunswick, N.J., 1963), p. 11. John Burrow, *Evolution and anthropology in the 1860's: The Anthropological Society of London, 1863–71*, Victorian Studies 7 (December 1963): 151.

6. Frances Power Cobbe, *Hereditary piety*, Theological Review (April 1870); reprinted in Cobbe, *Darwinism in Morals and Other Essays* (London, 1872), p. 36.

7. [Merivale], *Hereditary Genius*, p. 101.

8. David Hartley, *Observations on Man, His Frame, His Duty, and His Expectations*, 2 vols. (London, 1749).

9. See, for example, Henry Holland, "Hereditary Disease," in his *Medical Notes and Reflections* (London, 1839), pp. 18–25, or O. S. Fowler, *Hereditary Descent: Its Laws and Facts Illustrated and Applied to the Improvement of Mankind* (New York, 1840).

10. On the position of Gall and Spurzheim with regard to the hereditarian-environmentalist debate see, Owsei Temkin, *Gall and the phrenological movement,* Bull. Hist. Med. 21 (1947): 275; David Bakan, *The influence of phrenology on American psychology,* J. Hist. Beh. Sci. 2 (1966): 200–21; Robert M. Young, *Mind Brain and Adaptation in the 19th Century* (Oxford 1970), chap. 1.

11. Young, *Mind Brain and Adaptation,* chap. 5.

12. John D. Davies, *Phrenology, Fad and Science, a 19th Century American Crusade* (New Haven, 1955).

13. [Anon.] *Heredity,* J. Science 12 (April 1875): 159.

14. Allen Thomson, "Generation," in R. B. Todd and William Bowman, *Cyclopaedia of Anatomy and Physiology* (London 1836–1859), p. 474.

15. Thomson, *Generation,* p. 471.

16. John C. Greene, *The Death of Adam* (Ames Iowa, 1959), esp. chaps. 5–8; John Burrow, *Evolution and Society: A Study in Victorian Social Theory* (Cambridge, 1966); George Stocking, *Race, Culture and Evolution: Essays in the History of Anthropology* (New York, 1968), esp. chap. 10.

17. Francis Galton, *Memories of My Life* (London, 1908), p. 310.

18. *LLL,* 2: 88.

19. August Weisman, *Uber die Vererbung* (Jena, 1883). See, Frederick Churchill, *August Weismann and a break from tradition,* J. Hist. Bio. 1 (1968): 91–112.

20. For this reason it is incorrect to give Galton priority in the discovery of the continuity of germplasm, as several historians have done: L. C. Dunn, *A Short History of Genetics* (New York, 1965), p. 38; Robert C. Olby, *Origins of Mendelism* (London, 1966), p. 70.

21. Conway Zirkle, *The early history of the idea of the inheritance of acquired characteristics and of pangenesis,* Trans. Am. Phil. So. n.s. 35 (1946): 91–151.

22. Peter J. Vorzimmer, *Charles Darwin: The Years of Controversy, The "Origin of Species" and its Critics, 1859–1882* (Philadelphia, 1970).

23. Francis Galton, *Regression toward mediocrity in hereditary stature,* J. Anthro. Inst. 14 (1885): 246–63, and *Natural Inheritance* (London, 1889), pp. 134–35. For the history of the notion of repeated halving see, Olby, *Origins of Mendelism,* p. 68.

24. *Memories,* pp. 316–18.

25. Walter Houghton, *The Victorian Frame of Mind* (New Haven, 1957), passim.

26. Frank Buckland, Jr., to Francis Galton, 31 May 1865; *GA.*

27. Walter Houghton, ed., *The Wellesley Index to Victorian Periodicals, 1824–1900* (Toronto, 1966), 1: 554–56.

28. See, Francis Galton to William Bateson, 12 January 1904; *LLL,* 3: 220.

29. Some of this information (on Galton's voting habits, his friends, and his religious inclinations) was given to my by Galton's nephew and occasional travelling companion, Frank Butler, in a private conversation, February 1967. The rest of the biographical summary given here is an amalgam of material in *LLL* and *Memories.*

30. *Memories,* p. 82.

31. Francis Galton, *English Men of Science: Their Nature and Nurture* (London, 1874), p. 218.

32. Eliot Slater, *Galton's heritage,* Eugenics Review 52 (1960): 91–103.

33. Francis Galton to his brother Darwin Galton, 23 February 1851; *LLL,* 1: 232.

34. Francis Galton, *Measure of fidget,* Nature 32 (1885): 174. Some of the devices that Galton used for surreptitious counting are in *GA.*

35. *LLL,* 4: 457. The experiments were conducted in February 1859.

36. *Memories,* p. 161.

37. *Memories,* pp. 161 and 185.

38. C. J. Anderssen to Francis Galton, July 1855; *GA.*

39. *Memories,* p. 161.

40. *LLL,* 1: 177. Galton had the poem published privately in Cambridge; the whole text is in *GA.*

41. Francis Galton to his sister Elizabeth Galton Wheler, n.d.; *GA.* The letter seems to be from

the period 1844–49; it was sent from Kirkwall, Orkney and in it Galton referred to the birth of Mrs. Wheler's daughter, Lucy, who was born during this period.

42. Francis Galton to his father, Samuel Tertius Galton, 1 July 1841; *LLL,* 1: 155.

43. See n. 29.

44. Webb. *Modern England* (New York, 1968), p. 279; Phillip Appleman, et al., *1859; Entering an Age of Crisis* (Bloomington, 1962).

45. Houghton, *Victorian Frame of Mind,* chap. 1; William L. Burn, *The Age of Equipoise* (New York and London, 1964); Basil Willey, *Nineteenth Century Studies: Coleridge to Matthew Arnold* (New York and London, 1949).

46. Ruskin, *Unto This Last* (London, 1862), p. 1.

47. Arnold, *Culture and Anarchy* (1869), ed. J. Dover Wilson (Cambridge, 1932), chap. 1.

48. *Hereditary Genius* (1869) reprinted (London, 1962), p. 56.

49. [Anon.] *Heredity,* J. Science 12 (April 1875): 166.

50. Henry W. Holland, *Heredity,* Atlantic Monthly 52 (1883): 449.

51. See n. 6.

52. Mill, *Principles of Political Economy* (London, 1848), 1: 390.

53. Galton's marginal notes will be discussed in more detail below; his copy of *Variations* is in *GA*.

54. Francis Galton, *Blood relationship,* Proc. Roy. Soc. 20 (1872): 394–402. The stirp theory is discussed in more detail below.

55. Francis Galton to Charles Darwin, 3 Nov. 1875; Charles Darwin to Francis Galton, 4 Nov. [1875]; Francis Darwin to Francis Galton, n.d.; Francis Galton to Charles Darwin, 5 Nov. 1875. All in *LLL,* 2: 182–184.

56. Francis Galton, *Feasible experiments on the possibility of transmitting acquired habits by means of inheritance,* Brit. Assoc. Rep. (1889): 620; Nature 40 (5 Oct. 1889): 610. This proposal indicates that Galton did not accept Weismann's disproof of the inheritance of acquired characteristics, a proof based on the non-inheritance of mutilations. Galton did not, however, explain the reasons for finding Weismann's work inconclusive.

57. Charles Darwin to Francis Galton, 4 Jan. [1873]; *LLL,* 2: 176.

58. [Anon.], *Galton's "Inquiries into Human Faculty,"* Saturday Review (26 May 1883): 668.

59. Several notebooks containing plans and thoughts about the establishment of eugenics are in *GA*.

60. Francis Galton, *The possible improvement of the human breed under the existing conditions of law and sentiment,* Nature 64 (1 Nov. 1901): 659–65; also in, *Annual Report of the Smithsonian Institution* (Washington, 1901), pp. 523–38 and Pop. Sci. Mon. 60 (Jan. 1902): 218–33.

61. Romanes, *Review of "Inquiries into Human Faculty,"* Nature 28 (31 May 1883): 97.

62. J. A. Froude, *Thomas Carlyle. A History of His Life in London, 1834–1881* (London, 1884), 1: 290–91. See Houghton, *The Victorian Frame of Mind,* chap. 3.

63. This is another part of the poem already cited, n. 40.

64. *Memories,* p. 88. See Galton's comments on Mohammedanism in, *On Mr. Stanley's recent expeditions,* Edinburgh Review 147 (Jan. 1878): 187.

65. See "Daniel Douglas Home," *D.N.B.* Also Katherine Porter, *Through a Glass Darkly: Spiritualism in the Browning Circle* (Lawrence, Kansas, 1958).

66. [Anon.], *Spiritualism and its evidences,* Westminster Review 147 (April 1872): 461.

67. Ibid.

68. Louisa Galton's annual record, *GA*.

69. Francis Galton to Charles Darwin, 28 March 1872; *LLL,* 2: 63. This is one of six letters that Galton wrote to Darwin about spiritualism, 28 March 1872–November 1872; *LLL,* 2: 62–66.

70. *LLL,* 2: 66–67.

71. Francis Galton to Charles Darwin, 24 December 1869, *LLL* 1: plate 2.

72. See *LLL,* 2: 425 for a manuscript note which Pearson dated c. 1892 and which he regarded as an expression of Galton's ideas about religion; also, *LLL,* 2: 257, 282; 3: 271; 4: 471–72.

73. *LLL,* 3: 271. The remark was made to Karl Pearson.

74. Francis Galton, *Statistical inquiries into the efficacy of prayer,* Fortnightly Review n.s. 12 (August 1872): 125–35.

75. The article created a storm of controversy in the *Spectator* (August and September 1872). It also led to the publication of a refutation by G. J. Romanes, *Christian Prayer and General Laws* (London 1874). Galton removed the article from *Inquiries into Human Faculty* when that book was reprinted in 1907; it was still repugnant to some of the younger members of his family.

76. Galton to his niece, Millicent Lethbridge, Sept. 1883; *LLL,* 4: 472.

77. Francis Galton, *Inquiries into Human Faculty* (London, 1883), p. 210.

78. Francis Galton to Francis Darwin, 22 Oct 1885; *LLL,* 2: Plate 12.

79. Francis Galton to George Howard Darwin, 30 Jan 1876; *LLL,* 2: 191.

80. *Memories,* p. 322.

81. Francis Galton, *Eugenics as a factor in religion,* Sociological Papers 2 (1905): 52–53.

82. Houghton, *The Victorian Frame of Mind,* pp. 45–54.

83. Oliver Wendell Holmes, as quoted by a correspondent in the *Shrewsbury Gazette* (1894). A church steeple collapsed in Shrewsbury, Charles Darwin's birthplace, just a week after a meeting had been held to discuss a memorial to him. A rash of articles and letters appeared in the local newspaper, some correspondents praising Darwin's work, others insisting that the collapse of the steeple indicated God's disapproval. A collection of clippings about this incident, including the one from which the quotation was taken, can be found in the *Charles Darwin Papers, Cambridge University Library,* 107/54.

84. Moncure Conway to Francis Galton, 27 April 1882; *LLL,* 4: 471. Conway was an American scholar, editor of the works of Thomas Paine.

85. *Hereditary talent and character,* p. 322.

86. *Hereditary Genius,* p. 428.

87. Ibid.

88. Ibid.

89. Darwin to Galton, congratulating him on the publication of *Tropical South Africa,* 24 July [1853]; *LLL,* 1: 240. Darwin to Galton about camping, 28 May [1855]; *GA.* Darwin to Galton, thanking him for having sent a copy of *The Art of Travel,* 10 January [1856]; *GA.* Darwin to Galton, asking for information about the domestication of animals in Africa, 4 February [1857]; *GA.* Galton to Darwin, commenting on the publication of the *Origin of Species,* 9 December 1859; *LLL,* 2: Plate 18.

90. Diaries for the years 1853, 1854, 1862, 1877 are in *GA,* Louisa Galton's annual record covers the years 1853–96.

91. Darwin to Galton, 24 July [1853]; *LLL,* 1: 240.

92. Darwin's copies of Galton's books are in the *Darwin Collection,* University Library Cambridge.

93. Galton to Darwin, 9 December 1859; *LLL,* 2: Plate 18.

94. Ibid. The list of notes has subsequently disappeared.

95. Galton's marginal notes are on p. 175 (about the struggle for survival), p. 206 ("unity of type is explained by unity of descent"), and p. 227 (about regularity in cells of the beehive). His calculation of rate of increase is on p. 64. His copy of the *Origin* was a first edition.

96. *Hereditary Genius,* p. 421.

97. This and all other papers relating to the Erasmus Darwin Memorial are in *GA.*

98. Charles Darwin to J. D. Hooker, [March 1860]; Francis Darwin, ed., *The Life and Letters of Charles Darwin* (reprint, New York, 1959), 1: 87.

99. Galton's copy of *The Variations of Animals and Plants Under Domestication,* 2 vols. (London 1868), a first edition, is in *GA.* Galton also took long-hand notes on *The Variations;* these are also in *GA.*

100. *Variations,* 2: 24.

101. Ibid.

102. *Variations,* 2: 82.

103. *Variations,* 2: 81.

104. *Variations,* 2: 386.

105. *Hereditary Genius,* chap. 3. Sec. 4.

106. *Hereditary Genius,* p. 426.

107. *Hereditary Genius*, p. 423.

108. Pearson makes the same point about Galton's metaphysical attraction to pangenesis, *LLL*, 2: 119.

109. Darwin to Galton, 23 December [1869]; *LLL*, 1: Plate 6.

110. Galton to Darwin, 11 December 1869; *LLL*, 2: 157. For some unexplained reason Galton did not mention the purpose of his experiments; he simply asked advice about procuring pure-bred albino rabbits for "some peculiar experiments that have occurred to me in breeding animals." Darwin discovered his intent soon enough.

111. Charles Darwin to Alphonse de Candolle, 18 January 1873; Frances Darwin, ed., *More Letters of Charles Darwin* (London, 1903), 1: 348. See also the correspondence between Huxley and Darwin, ibid., 301 and Leonard Huxley, ed., *The Life and Letters of Thomas Henry Huxley*, 2nd ed. (London, 1903), 1: 384–87.

112. Darwin to Hooker, [21 May 1868]; *More Letters of Charles Darwin*, 1: 303.

113. E. Romanes, ed., *The Life and Letters of George John Romanes*, 2nd. ed. (London, 1896), pp. 36–50. Also, *More Letters of Charles Darwin*, 1: 286.

114. *LLL*, 2: 157.

115. *LLL*, 2: 160.

116. *LLL*, 2: 161.

117. Francis Galton, *Experiments in pangenesis by breeding from rabbits of a pure variety, into whose circulation blood taken from other varieties had previously been largely transfused*, *Proc. Roy. Soc.* 29 (1870—71): 404.

118. Nature 6 (27 April 1871): 502.

119. *Variations*, 2: 379.

120. Francis Galton, *Reply to Mr. Darwin*, Nature 6 (4 May 1871): 5–6.

121. Darwin to Galton, 8 November [1872]; *LLL*, 2: 175.

122. Galton to Darwin, 15 November 1872; *LLL*, 2: 175.

123. Galton composed a list of the letters that were in his possession in 1896 (presumably to assist Francis Darwin in collecting his father's letters); all the letters on that list are presently in *GA* and most have been published in *LLL*.

124. Darwin to Galton, 28 May [1873]; *LLL*, 2: 179.

125. Galton to Darwin, 14 April 1875; *LLL*, 2: 180.

126. Francis Galton, *A theory of heredity*, Contemporary Review 27 (December 1875): 80–95; a revised version appeared in J. Roy. Anthro. Inst. 5 (1875): 325–48.

127. Darwin to Galton, 2 November 1875; *LLL*, 2: 181. The embryological theories in question were those of M. Balbiani, *Sur l'embryogénie de la puce*, Comptes Rend. Acad. Sci. Paris 431 (1875): 901–4.

128. For all the correspondence see, *LLL*, 2: 181–90.

129. Darwin said this in a letter to Galton, 4 January 1873; *LLL*, 2: 176.

130. *Variations*, 2: 358–73. Darwin included one other phenomenon, the occasional influence of a male directly upon the female with which he has mated. I have eliminated it here because it is more or less irrelevant to this discussion and was largely irrelevant to Darwin's.

131. Francis Galton, *Blood Relationship*, received by the Royal Society 7 May 1872, published in the *Proceedings*, 13 June 1872, (1872): 394–401.

132. Ibid., p. 396.

133. Ibid., p. 401.

134. Francis Galton, *Hereditary improvement*, Frasers 7 (1873) 116–30.

135. Francis Galton, *The history of twins as a criterion of the relative powers of nature and nurture*, J. Roy. Anthro. Inst. 4 (1874): 126–30.

136. Francis Galton, *English Men of Science: Their Nature and Nurture* (London, 1874).

137. *The history of twins . . .* , p. 406.

138. See n. 126.

139. The expression "structureless elements" had been criticized by James Clerk Maxwell. Maxwell said that "structureless germ" was a *non-sequitor*, because if germs were different from each other they had to have some sort of structure. See Maxwell's article, "Atom" in the 9th ed. of the *Encyclopedia Britannica* (1875).

140. Charles Darwin to Francis Galton, 7 November [1875]; *LLL*, 2: 187. Darwin marked his

copy of the paper to indicate the offensive passages and sent the copy back to Galton; this copy subsequently disappeared. The reprint of *A Theory of Heredity* which is in the *Darwin Reprint Collection* (#1046) is the later version.

141. Darwin listed eight objections in all: two others dealt with the causes of sexuality, and one with Galton's discussion of twins. In the absence of Darwin's marked copy the three remaining comments are too vague to be connected with Galton's text.

142. Letters between Charles Darwin and Francis Galton, 4 November 1875–22 December 1875; *LLL*, 2: 181–90.

143. *A theory of heredity*, J. Roy. Anthro. Inst., second paragraph p. 342 and first paragraph p. 343.

144. Ibid., pp. 332–33.

145. *Blood relationship*, p. 400.

146. See n. 19.

147. August Weismann to Francis Galton, 23 February 1889; *LLL*, 4: 340–41. See also August Weismann, "The Continuity of Germ-plasm as the Foundation of a Theory of Heredity," published in *Essays Upon Heredity and Kindred Biological Problems*, Edward B. Poulton, et al., trans. (Oxford, 1889), p. 172, n. 3.

148. *Natural Inheritance*, chap. 5.

149. L. A. J. Quételet (1796–1894) was the Astronomer-Royal of Belgium. His probabilistic study of human populations appeared in *Essai sur l'homme* (1836) which was translated into English as *Essay on Man* (Edinburgh, 1838). Benjamin Gould was an American physician who undertook a statistical study of soldiers during the American Civil War, *Investigations in the Military and Anthropological Statistics of American Soldiers*, Sanitary Memoirs of the War of the Rebellion (New York, 1869).

150. See, for example, the treatment of Galton in Robert C. Olby, *Origins of Mendelism* (London, 1966), pp. 70–83; L. C. Dunn, *A Short History of Genetics* (New York, 1965), pp. 37–39, and Eric Nordenskjold, *History of Biology* (New York, 1929), pp. 585–87.

151. For the added details see Ruth Schwartz Cowan, *Francis Galton's statistical ideas: the influence of eugenics*, Isis 63 (1972): 509–28, from which the following discussion is abstracted.

152. *Hereditary Genius*, Sec.1, chapters 2 and 3.

153. Francis Galton, *Proposed statistical scale*, J. Roy. Anthro. Inst. 4 (1874): 136–37, or Nature 9 (5 March 1874): 342; *Statistics by intercomparison and remarks on the laws of frequency of error*, Phil. Mag. 49 (Jan. 1875): 34; *Proposal to apply for anthropological statistics from schools*, J. Roy. Anthro. Inst. 3 (1873–74): 308–11.

154. Francis Galton, *Relative supplies from town and country families to the population of future generations*, J. Stat. Soc. Lond. 26 (1873): 19–26; *Marlborough School statistics*, J. Roy. Anthro. Inst. 4 (1874): 126–30; *On the height and weight of boys aged 14 in town and country schools*, J. Roy. Anthro. Inst. 5 (1876): 174–80.

155. Francis Galton, *Address to the Anthropological Section of the British Association*, Brit. Assoc. Rep. (1885): 1207; also in Nature 32 (24 Sept. 1885): 507.

156. Francis Galton, *Typical laws of heredity*, Proceedings of the Royal Institution 8 (9 Feb. 1877): 282–301. A copy of the diagram can be found in *LLL*, 4: 4; it comes from a notebook labeled *Royal Institution Lecture, GA*.

157. Francis Galton, *Regression toward mediocrity in hereditary stature*, J. Anthro. Inst. 15 (1885): 246–63, and *Natural Inheritance* (London, 1889), passim.

158. On Galton's difficulties with mathematics see, R. J. Swinburne, *Galton's Law—formulation and development*, Annals of Science 21 (1965): 15–31.

159. *Natural Inheritance*, pp. 101–2.

160. Ibid.

161. Francis Galton, *Address to the Anthropological Section of the British Association*, Nature 32 (24 Sept 1885): 509.

162. Francis Galton, *Presidential address to the Anthropological Institute*, J. Anthro. Inst. 19 (1888): 411.

163. The material below is abstracted from Ruth Schwartz Cowan, *Francis Galton's contribution to genetics*. J. Hist. Biol. 5 (1972): 389–412.

164. *Memories*, p. 288.

165. These conflicting definitions of variation were analyzed in Prosper Lucas, *Traité Philosophique et Physiologique de l'Hérédité* (Paris, 1847), I: 170–85.

166. On all these matters see, *Natural Inheritance,* passim.

167. See, William Bateson, *Materials for the Study of Variation* (London, 1894), pp. 36–43; Hugo de Vries, *The Mutation Theory* (1901–03), trans. J. B. Farmer and A. D. Darbishire (Chicago, 1909), I: 45–53, 135–42.

168. J. A. Thomson, *Heredity* (London, 1908), p. 13.

169. William Bateson, *Problems of heredity as a subject for horticultural investigation,* J. Roy. Hort. Soc. 25 (1900), as reprinted in Beatrice Bateson, ed., *William Bateson, Naturalist* (Cambridge, 1928), p. 172.

170. See Galton's letters to his family, *LLL,* 4; passim, and Edward Wheler-Galton's remarks, *LLL,* 4: 531.

171. Francis Galton to his sisters Emma Galton and Elizabeth Wheler, 15 Dec 1899; *LLL,* 4: 515.

172. See *LLL,* 4: 657–58 for citations for these papers.

173. Francis Galton to Millicent Lethbridge, 28 Oct 1905; *LLL,* 4: 551.

174. Francis Galton to Millicent Lethbridge, 3 Oct 1910; *LLL,* 4: 611. The manuscript of the utopian scheme has been printed in *LLL,* 3: 417–24.

175. Francis Galton, *Personal identification and description,* Nature 38 (21 June 1888): 202.

176. Francis Galton, *The patterns in thumb and finger marks,* Phil. Trans. 182b (1891): 1–23; Francis Galton, *Finger Prints* (London, 1892).

177. *Identification of Habitual Criminals Report* (Blue Book, 1893 c. 1763).

178. See, *Finger Prints,* chaps. 11, 12.

179. *LLL,* 3: 189–90.

180. *Finger Prints,* p. 196.

181. In his autobiography Galton devoted one paragraph to Mendel, remarking upon the coincidence of their birth years (1822) and upon Mendel's work habits (*Memories,* p. 308). Of Mendel's theory of hybridization, Galton had only this to say: "Mendel clearly showed that there were such things as alternative atomic characters of equal potency in descent. How far characters generally may be due to simple or to molecular characters more or less correlated together, has yet to be discovered" (Ibid.).

182. See n. 28; also other letters in *GA* which are not printed in *LLL.*

183. For example: *Natural Inheritance,* chap. 3: *Fingerprints,* chap. 13; *Discontinuity in evolution,* Mind 3 (1894): 362–72.

184. Francis Galton, *The distribution of prepotency,* Nature 58 (14 July 1898): 246–47.

185. *Discontinuity in evolution,* p. 372.

186. The literature on this dispute is now fairly extensive. See, William Provine, *The Origins of Theoretical Population Genetics* (Chicago, 1971); P. Froggatt and N. C. Nevin, *The 'law of ancestral heredity' and the Mendelian-ancestrian controversy in England, 1889–1906,* J. Med. Gen. 8 (1971): 1–36; B. J. Norton, *The biometric defense of Darwinism,* J. Hist. Bio. 6 (1973): 283–316; A. G. Cock, *William Bateson, Mendelism and biometry,* J. Hist. Bio. 6 (1973): 1–35.

187. The best biographical source for Weldon is Karl Pearson, *W. F. R. Weldon,* Biometrika 5 (1906): 1–50.

188. See letters from Weldon to Galton, 14 May 1890 and 29 October 1891; *LLL,* 3: 483–84. The results of Weldon's work, including the first correlation coefficients determined for organisms other than man, were published in Weldon, *The variations occurring in certain Decapod Crustacea,* I. Crangon vulgaris, Proc. Roy. Soc. 47 (1890): 445–53, and *On certain correlated variations in* Crangon vulgaris, Proc. Roy. Soc. 51 (1892): 2–21.

189. For biographical details on Pearson see Egon Pearson, *Karl Pearson,* Biometrika 28 (1936): 193–257; 29 (1938): 161–237.

190. See *LLL,* 4: passim.

191. Galton, *Discontinuity in evolution.*

192. Wm. Bateson to Eva Biggs: 7 July 1909; *LLL,* 3: 288.

193. Letter from Bateson to G. H. Fowler, 24 June 1906; cited in Coleman, *Wm. Bateson . . .,* p. 243.

194. Proc. Roy. Soc. 57 (1895): 360–82.

195. See letter from Francis Galton to W. F. R. Weldon, 17 Nov. 1896; *LLL,* 3: 127.

196. Karl Pearson to Francis Galton, 12 Feb 1897; *LLL,* 3: 127–28.

197. Francis Galton to Karl Pearson, 15 Feb 1897; *LLL,* 4: 501.

198. For the details of this incident see letters exchanged between Francis Galton and Karl Pearson, *LLL,* 3: 240–51, 282. The quotation is from Francis Galton, *Biometry,* Biometrika 1 (1901): 8. Pearson's disputed paper is *On the principle of homotyposis and its relation to heredity. . . ,* Phil. Trans. 197a (1901): 285–379.

199. Karl Pearson, *The Ethic of Free Thought* (London, 1888).

200. Delivered 19 Nov. 1900 in Newcastle. Published, along with several appendices as Karl Pearson, *National Life from the Standpoint of Science* (London, 1905).

201. Francis Galton to Karl Pearson, 7 Jan. 1901; *LLL,* 3: 241.

202. Ibid.

203. Karl Pearson to Francis Galton, 10 Jan. 1901, *LLL,* 3: 242–43.

204. Nature 64 (31 Oct. 1901): 659–65.

205. See n. 60.

206. Millicent Lethbridge to Karl Pearson, 2 Oct. 1911, describing the contents of Francis Galton's trunks of letters; *GA*.

207. *LLL,* 3: 235.

208. Francis Galton, "Our National Physique—Prospects of the British Race—Are We Degenerating?" *Daily Chronicle,* 29 July 1903.

209. An abridged version of the lecture is in Nature 70 (26 May 1904): 82. For the reaction of those attending see, *LLL,* 3: 259–60.

210. Francis Galton, *Probability—The Foundation of Eugenics* (Oxford, 1907).

211. Karl Pearson to Francis Galton, 20 June 1907; *LLL,* 3: 323.

212. *LLL,* 3: 343, 345. The first issue of Eugenics Review (1909) carried a forward by Galton.

213. Samuel Lynn Hynes, *The Edwardian Turn of Mind* (Princeton, 1968), chaps. 2–4.

214. Benjamin Kidd, *Social Evolution* (New York, 1894), pp. 6–7.

215. Francis Galton, *Presidential address,* J. Roy. Anthro. Inst. 19 (1888): 406.

Conceptual History

A Review of
FRANÇOIS JACOB, *La logique du vivant: une histoire de l'hérédité.*
Paris. Éditions Gallimard, 1970, 354 pp.
FRANÇOIS JACOB, *The Logic of Life, A History of Heredity.*
trans. Betty E. Spillmann. New York. Pantheon Books. 1973. viii 348 pp.

Frederic L. Holmes

François Jacob's *La logique du vivant* will deeply affect the teaching and writing of the history of biology. Its recent appearance in translation as *The Logic of Life* should now spread the impact it has already made more broadly among English-speaking students of the subject. The book is written by a man who has a commanding stature within biology itself, and who has also immersed himself in the classical biological texts of earlier epochs. With these complementary sources of experience, Professor Jacob has been able to view the history of biology with a combination of breadth and penetration that few people can match. Scanning thought about and investigations of biological problems from the sixteenth century to the present, Jacob achieves a rare blend of grand scope with precise, cogent summaries of the ideas of individual scientists of the past.

The book's subtitle, "Une histoire de l'hérédité," must be understood in a particular sense. This is not the tracing of a subspecialty within the history of biology, but an analysis of concepts concerned with all areas of what has since 1800 been subsumed under the term biology. It is, however, focused upon heredity viewed as controlling that process, reproduction, which is most basic and indispensable to the nature of living things. Jacob further justifies his orientation by asserting that the two traditional poles of biological thought—the view of living organisms as parts of a vast system covering the earth, and

---

Frederic L. Holmes, Department of History of Medicine and Science, University of Western Ontario.

the analysis of the systems that comprise each individual organism—"are joined together at the level of heredity." The validity of Jacob's perspective is borne out in the recurrent theme of the book, that concepts related to heredity in different historical periods were shaped by changes in the whole range of conceptions about organisms, and about the spatial and temporal relationships of organisms with other organisms.

Jacob has pursued his objectives with undeviating concentration. The book contains few biographical details concerning the scientists whose ideas he describes. There are no conventional accounts of great discoveries. He gives only brief and general, although highly penetrating, sketches of the methods of investigation utilized during successive epochs. Instead he firmly fixes his attention on the description of the *concepts* prevailing in the various areas of biological investigation, and on the distinctions between the ways in which successive epochs viewed problems related to living organisms. At this level his analyses are brilliantly incisive. Except for his description of the most recent periods, in which the historical dimension nearly disappears, Jacob treats material that is already familiar to most historians of biology. He deals almost entirely with the well-known works of figures who are already regarded as outstanding spokesmen of their respective times. Yet in his cogent restatements of their views, in the juxtapositions, comparisons, and contrasts he provides of the concepts representative of successive stages of biological thought, Jacob has attained a fresh and revealing perspective on the whole subject. Seldom have the distinguishing features of the biological concepts of different historical periods been so sharply delineated and the demarcations between them so clearly isolated.

I can mention here only a few of the most general of the remarkably rich array of themes that Jacob's spare, succinct style has packed into a book of moderate length. Up until the end of the sixteenth century, according to him, no concept of a species as a stable series of visible forms linked by generation could exist, because living organisms were connected to the other objects of the world by a heterogenous mixture of similarities, signs, and hidden meanings. The production of a new being was not a natural process, but an individual act of divine creation, a generation rather than a reproduction. With the seventeenth century, the nature of knowledge itself changed; no longer involved in the tracing of networks of analogies and signs, knowledge became concerned only with observing and establishing connections between visible phenomena. During the "classical age,"which extended until near the end of the eighteenth century, generation became the expression of a regular law; but the requirement that any theory be compatible with the mechanistic philosophy, together with the condition that all explanations during that period were based on "visible structures," made the doctrine of preformation and preexistence the only acceptable theory of generation. The study of living things followed two streams, that of physiology and of natural history. The first was dependent on the application of concepts available from mechanics and chemistry, because there was no conception of living beings as distinct from other physical objects. Natural history rested upon the concept of the species as a permanent entity, defined by a set of visible characters, the individuals linked by chains of generation. Preformation harmonized well with this view, because, if all the "germs" of successive generations of plants and animals existed within their ancestors from the first creation, then there could be no historical development, no changes of character resulting from time and circumstances. Preformation was undermined during the eighteenth century by studies of regeneration, hybridization, and inheritance of unusual characteristics that were found to be transmitted equally through male and female parents. The prevailing conceptions of living beings, however, did not permit the replacement of the doctrine by an epigenetic view of generation. The attempts of Maupertuis and of Buffon to describe generation as the aggregation of organic molecules were not successful, but did represent recognition of the basic problem that any explanation based on the assemblage of elementary units must face; the necessity for a "memory" to guide the process. It was that problem that Buffon tried to solve with his difficult idea of the "moule intérieur." It was he who first applied the idea of *reproduction* to the general process of development of successive generations.

Near the end of the eighteenth century, Jacob asserts, a profound change occurred in the way in which living organisms were perceived. Beneath the visible order of their surface characters there emerged a conception of hidden relations constituting an internal organization. The idea of organization established for the first time a sharp distinction between living beings and inorganic things. A new science, biology, appeared, having as its object of analysis "no longer visible structure, but organization."

In physiology Jacob associates the recognition of a "hidden architecture" particularly with Lavoisier, who saw that the function of respiration involves a series of associated processes, including digestion and absorption to replace the oxidized substances, excretions, and adjustments of the temperature. The connections between these operations required in turn that the organs within which they occur be interdependent, organized into coordinated systems. At the same time, with Vicq-d'Azyr and Cuvier, naturalists began to classify animals on the basis of their internal anatomy rather than their surface features, to define major groups according to their general plans of organization, and to turn zoology into an analysis of comparative functions.

At the beginning of the nineteenth century the plan of organization was a coordinated arrangement of organs. By mid-century the cell theory had identified a whole new level of organization that not only provided a structural unity applicable to all living beings, but reordered all other conceptions of organisms and of their interrelations. ''That which was most profoundly convulsed by the cell theory,'' Jacob believes, ''was the study of the reproduction of living beings.'' Already microscopic observations of spermatozoa and ova, and the embryological studies of von Baer and others, had laid to rest the old view that generation could be the growth of a preformed individual; reproduction was truly a ''new construction at each birth in the series of generations.'' The cell theory showed, however, that at the origin of this development there is a unit that has ''an architecture which already possesses all of the attributes of life.'' In its simplest form reproduction consists of the multiplication of such units.

A series of conceptual shifts that took place between the late eighteenth and early nineteenth centuries were essential prerequisites, Jacob argues, for the evolutionary theories of Darwin and Wallace. According to Jacob none of the eighteenth-century ''precursors'' of evolution held truly evolutionary views. One reason they could not was the eighteenth-century view of nature as a continuous chain of all possible forms of living beings. There were no sensible gaps between each species and those that most closely resembled it. Even Lamarck believed that species were transformed only into the other species comprising the fixed, uninterrupted order of nature. ''That which radically separated all earlier evolutionary thought from that of Darwin and Wallace, was the notion of contingency applied to living beings.'' The three crucial conceptions necessary in order to view species as the contingent outcomes of their previous history derived, Jacob believes, from the work of Cuvier. His division of animals into *embranchements* based on different plans of organization broke the continuity of living forms, showing that the major groups were dispersed and isolated from each other. His paleontological discoveries demonstrated that during successive geological epochs groups of species disappeared and were replaced by modified forms. His belief that the superficial, visible characters differentiating closely related animals can vary without affecting their functional organizations created a place for the idea of fortuitous variations.

In his remarkably lucid description of the structure of Darwin's evolutionary views, Jacob stresses that although Darwin did not use mathematical treatments, his attitude toward variations was similar to that which produced statistical mechanics during the same era. He thought always in terms of populations; one could not specify the nature or effects of any individual variation, but with large numbers the small advantages conferred on certain individuals produced the inevitable consequences of natural selection. This feature of Darwin's thought links him with Boltzmann and Gibbs in physics, and with Mendel's handling of heredity, as manifestations of a radical change ''in the very manner of considering objects,'' which appeared at the middle of the century. Jacob follows the consequences of this new view, particularly for the emergence of the concept of the gene, a purely statistical entity that "transformed the representation of the living world."

Classical genetics was, Jacob points out, a "black box" subject. It did not attempt to establish the connections between the external character and the invisible, abstract gene that controlled it and did not elucidate the mechanism by which the gene gives expression to the character. The study of such connections required the merger of two sciences, that which had dealt statistically with "the unit of heredity," and that which had dealt chemically with "the unit of execution," the enzyme. To prepare for his discussion of that synthesis Jacob sketches out the development of organic chemistry and of concepts of fermentation during the nineteenth century, and the development during the twentieth of techniques such as chromatography, x-ray crystallography, and the use of isotopes, which made it possible to bring together the study of genes and enzymes at the molecular level. In considerably greater detail he shows how the success of this synthesis depended on the choice of the simplest system in which the overall process could be investigated, that of bacterial cells.

Despite his attention to the prerequisite methods, Jacob views the new molecular biology as fundamentally the result of another broad conceptual departure. It is, he says, "the concept of information which, at the middle of the present century made this order and its transmission accessible to analysis." The concept of genes as containing *programs* that are translated and carried out within the cells is, in his view, what most clearly differentiates the current epoch in biology from the earlier period. The concept of a program has also brought about the disappearance of both the old vitalism and the old reductionism. The last quarter of the book is an exposition of contemporary views of living organisms based on this fundamental idea. Jacob appears to have changed his approach considerably in this section. In earlier chapters he analyzed the conceptions of older biologists in order to show how their views were conditioned by the structures of thought of their epochs. In this section he appears to be describing organisms as they "really are." Yet he brings himself back at the very end with the conclusion that "Today everything is messages, codes, information. What dissection in the future will dislocate our objects to reconstitute them in some new space?" If the statement is more than rhetoric, Jacob is suggesting that the present biological era is merely one more in the series of epochs he has delineated, fated like its predecessors to end through some fundamental conceptual rupture.

This cursory sampling of the topics treated by Jacob illustrates also two of his central concerns. Repeatedly he stresses that the solutions possible for any given biological problem during a given epoch were determined by the whole set of conceptions about organisms prevailing at the time. The existing point of view, he believes, is a more basic limiting factor even than the range of investigative techniques available. Second, he seeks to identify the very broad changes in the nature of "knowledge" itself that have caused parallel shifts in the approaches to specific problems in several areas of biology or of science at large. Similarly, he focuses on the effects of changes in one area of biological investigation on other areas. Historians of science commonly espouse such objectives, but few are as effective as Jacob in unraveling linkages which are at the same time specific and far-reaching. In most instances Jacob is persuasive in his delineations of such interactions. Occasionally, however, his committment to this approach, together with his method of establishing connections through the conceptual analysis of texts rather than by tracing historical influences, misleads him. Thus, among the developments necessary to the view that living organisms are products of contingent events, and therefore part of the radical shift in thought prerequisite to Darwinian evolution, he argues, was the emergence of the cell theory. The cell theory provided a conception of ontogeny in which different organisms developed in analogous ways, but did not follow a common path determined by "necessity." This logically persuasive relation between cell theory and evolutionary theory could not have been historically operative, however, because Darwin conceived of the central features of his theory during the same years that Schleiden and Schwann were reaching their generalizations about cells, well before the cell theory had permeated biological thought. Even in the *Origin of Species* Darwin took little account of the cellular organization of organisms.

Jacob's image of the history of biology as composed of homogenous epochs dominated by particular conceptual assemblages—discrete periods separated from the past and future by abrupt *"bouleversements"*—offers a highly suggestive, and I believe, fruitful means to organize one's view of the subject and to fit complex developments into clear patterns. Yet it appears to me that the divisions and thresholds he has demarcated are in part artificial, drawn as much from Jacob's own point of view as from the web of history itself. Repeatedly, he describes such transformations in stark declarations, such as: "The generation of a being changed its role and status (p. 73)"; "what was transformed at the beginning of the 19th century was thus the manner in which living beings are arranged in space (p. 126)"; "the method of statistical analysis transformed biology into a quantitative science (p. 220)"; "it was the entire representation of living beings which was thus upset (p. 227)"; "It was the entire manner of regarding heredity which was thus upset (p. 236)"; (the English edition softens this claim somewhat, to "The way of looking at heredity was thus radically transformed"); and, "In a few years the theory of the gene had transformed the representation of the living world (p. 245)." Jacob is precise about the conceptual reconstructions involved in these transformations, but notably vague about how and when the new conceptions spread through communities of biologists. Sometimes he says that such a process occurred gradually, or over a few years, but at other times he merely states that "the eighteenth century," or "the early nineteenth century" viewed a situation differently from the preceding or succeeding age. Correspondingly, Jacob portrays the epochs reaching from one such transition to the next as relatively uniform. He does describe divergent approaches such as those of the "systematists" and "methodists" in eighteenth-century taxonomy, or the debate between Cuvier and Geoffroy Saint-Hilaire over whether there is a common plan of organization for all animals. These appear, however, as variations on a common theme rather than as deep conflicts. Jacob's perspective is important, suggesting that what have often been described as fundamental issues took place actually at a superficial level compared to the assumptions shared by both sides through their common participation in the conceptual configuration of their epochs. Yet I believe that, as with the case of the ruptures, Jacob has assumed rather than established that within each of his periods a general consensus reigned concerning the concepts involved.

Both the homogeneities and the discontinuities seem to me in part products of Jacob's method of reconstructing the conceptual structures of the past. Except for the twentieth century, which is almost nameless in his description, he examines each period by analyzing texts written by several well-known individuals he regards as representative. For the pre-seventeenth-century era, for example, he utilizes chiefly the writings of Paré, Cardan, Fernel, Aldrovandi, Belon, Paracelsus, and Cesalpino. Eighteenth-century views are drawn largely from Bonnet, Maupertuis, Buffon, Réaumur, and Haller. After summarizing the ideas of such people, usually with some well-selected quotations included, Jacob identifies the points of view that emerge with those of the "age" as a whole. Sometimes he relies for his exposition of a major topic on the views of a single scientist, as when he equates the entire nineteenth-century foundation of experimental physiology with the personal synthesis of Claude Bernard, or associates the application of chemistry to vital phenomena in the mid-nineteenth century with Justus Liebig's "animal chemistry," and elucidates the origin of a general synthetic organic chemistry mainly from Marcelin Berthelot's *La Synthèse chimique*. In thus leaping from the writings of a few major figures, who most fully espoused a certain point of view, to the defining characteristics of an epoch, Jacob naturally risks imparting the appearance of greater uniformity than actually existed. Physiologists contemporary with Bernard did not all conform to his ideal view of the field; and as many opposed as followed Liebig's way of applying chemistry to physiology. If a broader spectrum of writers had been covered in the discussion of each topic, I believe that the resulting pictures would reveal considerably more heterogeneity—countercurrents of various types, competing schools, writers in one epoch maintaining views supposed to have been characteristic of an earlier or later epoch. The epochs would appear less discrete, interpenetrating each other to such a degree that some of the boundaries Jacob delineates would seem more like useful logical abstractions than indicators of real historical convulsions.

Jacob's identification of the views of an age with those of influential individuals is not attributable exclusively to his method of historical analysis, for he seems really to believe that in former ages the major turning points in the history of biology were largely the achievements of a few outstanding men. Thus he is able to write, "It is with the work of Virchow, of Darwin, of Claude Bernard, of Mendel, of Pasteur, of Berthelot that the concepts, methods, the objects of study which are the source of modern biology were defined." In striking contrast, he describes the biology of the twentieth century in terms of anonymous concepts and methods. Perhaps he justifies this disparity in his approach by the changing scale of biological investigation. In the introduction he writes, "The importance of the . . . individual decreases in proportion as the number who practice the science increase." It is hard to understand how Jacob, with the deep understanding he has shown of the writings of those enumerated in the above passage, could be as unaware as he seems to be of the fact that the biology of their time already involved large numbers of people; and that the concepts out of which modern biology developed were the fruits of the collective efforts of many others besides these few giants.

La logique du vivant scrupulously cites the primary sources on which it draws, but contains scarcely any references to secondary sources. This is unfortunate. Despite his originality in the use of primary texts, Jacob has inevitably obtained much of his extensive knowledge of the history of science from other historians, and it would be helpful to know upon whom he has relied. Even without references it seems evident from the pervasive resemblances between the book and the writings of Michel Foucault that Jacob must have found much of the inspiration for his project in the work of his colleague at the Collège de France. Jacob's general approach, in fact, can be viewed as an application of some of the types of analysis Foucault has advocated in *L'archéologie du savoir.* According to Foucault, one should analyze discourses that have come down to us in written texts, dissecting, explaining, making explicit the connections between statements, comparing alternative choices made by different authors within the boundaries permitted by the conceptual structure of the epoch, but one should not search for the silent thoughts of the author, or the origins of his ideas, which lie inaccessible behind the text. One should, Foucault writes, seek to elucidate "relations of statements to one another (even if they escape the consciousness of the author)." Jacob's work accords well with these mandates. He is concerned exclusively with the meaning of the written texts of the scientists whose writings he analyzes, usually saying nothing about their careers, the chronological development of their views, or the personal origins of the positions they took. He analyzes their views as coherent systems, with little regard for changes in the opinions an individual held during his lifetime. Jacob also makes little distinction between implications of particular concepts that were evident to the authors, and implications that he himself can discern from the perspective of later events but that were probably not visible at the time. Foucault stressed the importance of defining not only the unities of discourse, the "'epochs' or 'centuries',"" by delineating the stable assemblages of concepts that unify them but also the "ruptures," and "interruptions" that separate one epoch from another. Such patterns, as we have seen, permeate Jacob's treatment.

These resemblances may not in themselves demonstrate a direct influence of Foucault's program on Jacob's endeavor, for both Foucault and Jacob may share a mode of discourse within current French historiography that my own distance from that intellectual community prevents me from seeing. There are in addition, however, resemblances between *La logique du savòir* and Foucault's *Les mots et les choses* that are too specific to be mistaken. Jacob's account of the transformation of the nature of knowledge between the sixteenth and seventeenth centuries, and the manifestations of that change in natural history; his description of the characteristics of the "classical age"; his arguments against the existence of true evolutionary concepts during the eighteenth century; his account of the shift from "visible structures" to "internal organization" as the basis for describing and classifying organisms and as the precondition for the origin of *biology* as the study of life; his attribution to Cuvier of a central role in the development of the idea of contingency in nature; and a number of related topics, are so similar to Foucault's discussions that there must be real connections between the two books.

In none of these instances does Jacob merely reiterate Foucault's discussion. Rather he adopts the conclusions for a considerably different purpose. Foucault treated the transition from the natural history of the "classical age" to the biology of the early nineteenth century as one of three parallel shifts in different fields of thought, together revealing a more basic transformation in the underlying "episteme" that sets the conditions under which thought about any special organized subject is possible. Jacob, on the other hand, is describing the history of biology itself and stresses the effects of general shifts of view as they affect various fields within that science. Jacob's borrowing of concepts which Foucault had derived from one set of problems to use in the description of another partially overlapping set, however, has created some difficulties, of which Jacob is apparently not aware. Foucault's description of the change is based on a comparison of eighteenth-century taxonomical texts with their counterparts of the early nineteenth century. Within this context he can argue convincingly that the concept of internal organization became the "foundation of the order of nature" only at the end of the eighteenth century, with the work of de Jussieu, Vicq d'Azyr, and Lamarck. Jacob, however, applies the same idea to other areas of biology as well—to theories of generation, to ideas about the elementary units comprising organic structure, and to physiology. As we have seen, he credits Lavoisier with the recognition of a total organization of the organs of the body into systems subservient to the "grand functions." According to Jacob, by then "It was no longer possible to consider the lungs or the stomach, the heart or the kidneys independently. A body . . . is a whole of which the parts depend upon one another and of which each fills a particular function in the general interest." This extension of Foucault's doctrine is, however, untenable. The concept that organs are interconnected in functional systems is at least as old as Aristotle's description of the heart and blood vessels as a system serving the general functions of nutrition and sensation. By the time of Galen most of the conspicuous organs of the body had been integrated into several functional systems—the stomach, intestines, and portal veins as the means of delivering and concocting food; the liver and veins as a nutritive system (served also by the spleen, bile duct, and kidneys, which removed impurities); the heart and arteries as the system that distributed heat and pneuma; and the sense organs, brain, nerves, and muscles as the system through which sensations and motions are integrated. Although particular organizational arrangements were substantially modified by such later events as the discovery of the circulation, the general conception of a functional organization of internal organs was never lost. The naturalists whom Foucault treats did not originate the concept of internal organization, but adapted it from traditional anatomy and physiology, began for the first time to *compare* systematically the organizations of different classes of plants and animals and used the results as a basis for the reform of classificatory systems. Thus the boundary which in Jacob's view separates all areas of nineteenth-century biology from the corresponding areas in previous ages is actually less comprehensive than he makes it out to be.

One could raise similar questions concerning the scope and significance of some of the other conceptual thresholds Jacob has identified. In doing so, however, one would at the same time underline the boldness and sweep of his venture. Closer examination will undoubtedly show that his epochs are sometimes less cohesive, and their separation less sharp, than he has portrayed them, but this is not likely to obliterate them. He has surveyed a vast terrain from a great height, but with a sharp and telescopic eye; his book should for a long time provide stimulation, guidance, and provocation to those of us who plod in a more mundane fashion along the ground.

THE JOHNS HOPKINS UNIVERSITY PRESS

This book was composed in VIP Times Roman text and display type by The Composing Room from a design by Susan Bishop. It was printed and bound by Publication Press, Inc.